CHILDHOOD
INJURY

Jack G. Shiller, M.D., is also the author of
Childhood Illness

CHILDHOOD INJURY

A Common Sense Approach

Jack G. Shiller, M.D.

Illustrations by Neil O. Hardy

𝔰𝔇

Stein and Day/*Publishers*/New York

To Rustin McIntosh,
who taught me how to think,
and
to Bill Silverman,
who taught me how to question

First published in 1977
Copyright © 1977 by Jack G. Shiller
All rights reserved
Printed in the United States of America
Stein and Day/*Publishers*/Scarborough House,
Briarcliff Manor, N.Y. 10510

Pages 13 and 14 of "Your Child and Household Safety," by Jay M. Arena,
M.D., reprinted by permission of the publisher, Chemical Specialities
Manufacturers Association, Inc.

Library of Congress Cataloging in Publication Data

Shiller, Jack G.
    Childhood injury.

    Includes index.
    1. Children—Wounds and injuries. 2. Medicine,
Popular. I. Title. [DNLM: 1. Wounds and
injuries—In infancy & childhood—Popular works.
W0700 S556c]
RD93.5.C4S52   617′.1   76-41839
ISBN 0-8128-2066-5

Contents

LIST OF ILLUSTRATIONS

Introduction

Courage and reason often disappear in the most courageous and reasonable parents when they are suddenly faced with an injured child. It may ever have been thus, but I doubt it, for many "modern" influences have modified our attitudes.

Our child-oriented society places an unprecedented premium on the health and welfare of little ones. And our mind's eye pictures these children as healthy, whole, unscarred. Thus when there's a possibility that serious injury has occurred, panic ensues. The panic usually takes the form of a hurried trip to the doctor's office or local hospital emergency room, frequently by ambulance, without any attempt at evaluation of the seriousness of the problem.

Many children are *needlessly* brought to the doctor or emergency room after relatively minor physical trauma. Their parents "just want to make sure" or "will sleep better knowing that someone has seen the child." After all, they "can't afford to take any chances!"

The word "afford" is important here, because many families have health insurance, and don't even have to pay for the visit. Almost all health insurance covers emergency visits to the doctor's office or hospital emergency room. But these visits, often an unnecessary luxury, create such a demand for service that their cost is being priced out of the realm of reasonable medical expense.

And then the phenomenon I call "malpractice medicine" takes over. Physicians may order x rays, laboratory tests or even consultations from other physicians, not necessarily on good clinical grounds but defensively, in case the patient is unhappy with his medical care or decides to sue after unforeseen complications occur. This "legal defensive medicine" is fostered by police officers, ambulance attendants and even bystanders who, anticipating legal action in even the most minor traffic accidents, will urge people to be "checked" by their physicians "just to be sure."

All of these niceties cost money and help to drive up the cost of medical care. Ever-increasing insurance premiums, the need for expanded emergency room facilities and unnecessary private physician's bills must all be paid for.

It is the purpose of this book to educate parents and others taking care of children in the *evaluation* of the injured child, and in the subsequent care of that child when professional help is NOT required.

How does a parent know when it is and when it isn't? That's what the book is all about. Every cut or laceration does *not* require stitches, every head injury does *not* require skull x rays, and every injury to an arm or leg does *not* require a cast, sling, or crutches!

As in my earlier book, *Childhood Illness,* I have begun with a chapter on general considerations. In subsequent chapters various types of injury are treated in the order in which they occur most frequently. Because of the subject matter, this follows an anatomical classification which should be helpful for easy reference.

At the outset, however, let it be clear that this book is not an attempt to compete with standard first-aid manuals. The American Red Cross has an excellent one which, in its first edition (1973), is a broadened and revised update of the standard reference first-aid manual it has been publishing for 50 years. In such a manual one learns what to do for an injured person—usually—*until* one can get competent medical care.

Further, this is not a do-it-yourself book on the treatment of injuries that *should* receive professional help. In no way do I wish to suggest that good medical care should be denied any patient *when that care is appropriate.* Rather, let me try to explain when such care is necessary, and when it is not, and what remedies or treatments may be helpful.

One will find many types of injuries in this book that are either unique to children or most infrequently seen in adults. To the best of my knowledge this information has never been published for lay consumption and will therefore be dealt with rather fully. Conversely, there will be many injuries commonly referred to in first-aid manuals that ordinarily do not occur in children and which therefore will not be considered.

Many parents have told me that they found *Childhood Illness* most useful when they familiarized themselves with the contents initially, and then consulted it for specifics when the occasion demanded. This should also be the case for *Childhood Injury.*

Throughout the book the child has been referred to as "he" to circumvent the cumbersome use of "he or she" for each description.

Once again I acknowledge with deep gratitude the help and advice of Bob Appleby, Mal Beinfield and Dean Martin who reviewed the manuscript, Neil Hardy whose illustrative insight never ceases to amaze me, and Angela Miller and all the Stein and Day people who continue to put up with me.

Medical care, like energy, must be conserved if it is to be available and affordable when it is really needed. If this book helps parents to deal wisely with their children's injuries, and in so doing fosters their self-confidence, then it will have served its intended purpose.

1

The Injured Child

GENERAL CONSIDERATIONS

Parental reactions of fear—even panic—over many injuries are really unreasonable when one considers the number of children who are injured every minute of every day. Most of these injuries are minor, *not* life threatening. The lump on the head, bruise, cut or sprained ankle could not be termed horrendous traumas. Yet they frequently evoke an uncertainty about proper medical care and that leads to feelings of anxiety, fear, and then an unnecessary visit to the doctor or emergency room.

Let us take a look at the injured child, and try to understand what's happening to him. What does he feel? How does he react? Is he in trouble? How can we tell? What should we do?

There's an old adage that applies particularly to pediatric problems: "Don't just *do* something, stand there!" No, we haven't written that incorrectly. It means,

"Don't be in such a rush to *do* something. Stand back and evaluate the situation." Frequently a minute or two spent in observation and evaluation will clarify the problem, alleviate the panic and make attempts at help more intelligent.

GENERAL BEHAVIOR AND APPEARANCE

The injured child is frightened. Invariably there has been some sudden, often violent movement, either of the child or something around him, that caused the accident. This is frightening. Now, suddenly, he hurts! This too is frightening. The people around him show fear and panic in their faces. This is frightening. There may be blood, and this will frighten both the youngster and his parent.

Crying and Breath Holding

Most often the child will begin to cry lustily. This should be the first encouraging sign! A child who can cry with vigor has probably not injured the vital organs in his chest or neck, and that's a plus! A child who is crying forcefully may be allowed to continue crying for a minute or two while you ascertain the location and extent of the injury.

Sometimes an older infant or toddler will begin to cry, and prolong the first sound of crying for so long that he turns dusky blue and may even pass out. This is *breath holding,* and is quite harmless. If the child does pass out, normal breathing will resume immediately. Color returns to normal as soon as breathing starts again, and consciousness returns within a few seconds.

The only significance of this event is that it must be differentiated from unconsciousness due to the injury itself. Children who hold their breaths usually cry first. The child struck unconscious from a head injury will usually *not* cry first.

The Visceral Reaction

Many children don't cry. One might almost say they are dumbfounded by the accident and forget to cry. In this situation a "visceral" reaction frequently takes place, in which the external blood vessels of the skin constrict, forcing blood into the deep or "visceral" organs of the body. This produces paleness. At the same time the child may break out into a cold sweat, and a concurrent sudden nausea will make the victim look almost green. They usually do not vomit, though they may.

These signs of a visceral reaction are the same as those seen with "shock" caused by blood loss. (Actually, the mechanism is the same. In the visceral reaction blood is "lost" from the rest of the body into the visceral organs.) However, since there is no real blood loss, the signs disappear quickly as blood is redistributed back into the rest of the body. "Shock" will be discussed in the next section.

WHEN TO GET HELP FAST—DON'T THINK, CALL!

If a child is seriously injured, help must be summoned immediately. But how can you tell how urgent or critical the problem is? Here are three situations in which no doubt exists. GET HELP FAST!

Loss of Consciousness

1. Send for help
2. Don't move the patient
3. Ensure adequate breathing (see below)
4. Control bleeding
5. Keep the patient warm

This usually implies a head injury of relatively serious nature. How serious will be determined later. The best position is supine (flat on his back). Move the child as little as possible to attain this. (He can't tell you what hurts, and you might do more harm than good.) Elevate the chin slightly to ensure an adequate airway, and hold the tongue if it keeps falling to the back of the throat. (Fig. 1-1) It will be less inclined to slip out of your fingers if you grasp it in a piece of cloth.

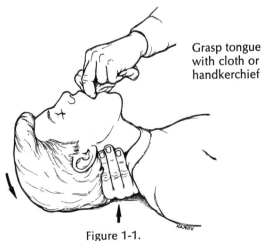

Grasp tongue with cloth or handkerchief

Figure 1-1.

Some children who lose consciousness have convulsions for a minute or two. If this happens, use a bite stick (toothbrush handle or stick wrapped with a piece of cloth) to keep him from biting his tongue. (Fig. 1-2) The wrapping will prevent broken teeth. Stop the bleeding if present (see below). Keep him warm and wait for help.

Many seriously injured children vomit. Be prepared to turn the patient's head to the side to clear the mouth of vomited material before it is sucked down into the windpipe.

Difficulty in Breathing

1. Send for help
2. Elevate chin
3. Examine mouth and throat for foreign material (gum, toy, etc.)
4. Choking treatment (see p. 27)
5. Secure tongue
6. Remove mucus and secretions
7. Artificial resuscitation if necessary

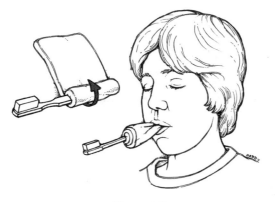

Figure 1-2.

Respirations are adequate when breathing is *not* labored and skin color is normal. Dusky or bluish skin color implies lack of oxygen. Noisy, irregular breathing sounds like obstruction to the airway. Vomitus, mucus or secretions in the mouth or throat will make a gurgling noise. Elevation of the chin may cure most of this. The mouth and back of the throat should be examined for chewing gum, lollipop sticks, small toys or anything else commonly found in children's mouths. This is best done carefully with your finger, rather than trying to see in there. Hold a small child upside down. Bend a larger child forward when you do this, *so as not to push a foreign object further down.*

If choking is suspected, the small child should be turned upside down and struck sharply between the shoulder blades. Larger children may be half-jackknifed off the end of a bed, table or counter top and struck similarly (Fig. 1-3).

The older child might benefit from the Heimlich Maneuver. Grab him from behind, around the upper midriff—lower chest area—lock your wrists (or hold one wrist with the other hand) and give a short sharp yank! This is intended to elevate the diaphragm, compress the chest and explosively force a foreign body out of the windpipe. (See Fig. 1-4)

It should be noted that as of this writing the Heimlich Maneuver is still being discussed in the medical literature, and has not been recommended for use in choking children. This is because their chest cages may be too fragile, and other nearby organs too delicate to withstand sudden, sharp pressure. But in a life-threatening situation, especially in older children, I believe the trial is justified.

The supine patient with an elevated chin may have

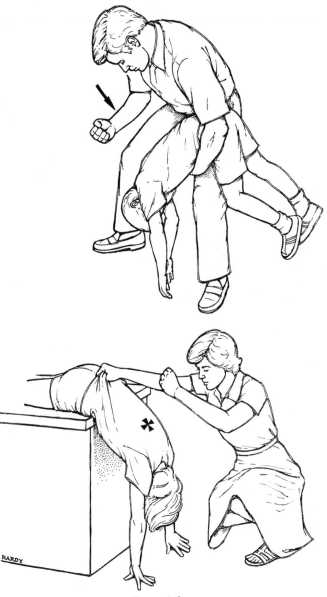

Figure 1-3.

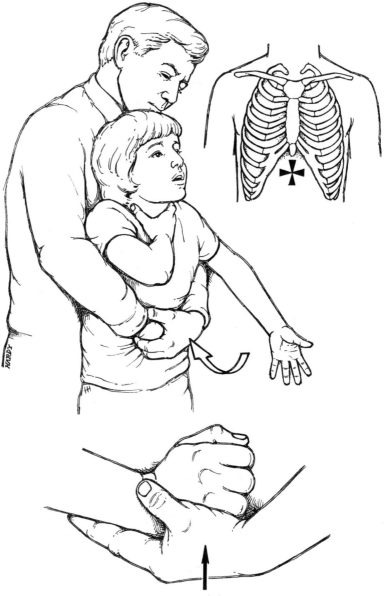

Figure 1-4.

difficulty keeping his tongue from flopping into the back of his throat. It may have to be held for him. Again, the cloth or handkerchief-wrapped tongue is less slippery and easier to hold.

As mentioned above, a child who is having difficulty breathing because of convulsions will need a bite stick (handkerchief-wrapped toothbrush handle or the like) inserted in the side of his mouth between his upper and lower back teeth to keep him from biting his tongue. It must be remembered that all these efforts are being directed at maintaining a clear airway.

Mucus, saliva and other secretions may have to be removed from the mouth occasionally. This is best done with your index finger wrapped in cloth or a handkerchief.

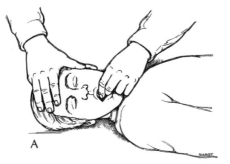

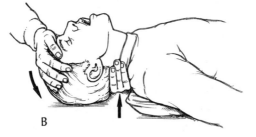

Figure 1-5A.

The odds are you won't have suction available. Finally, artificial respiration may be necessary. (See Fig. 1-5 and Chapter 14) The mouth-to-mouth method is easiest, most readily remembered and probably most effective. Remember that you're going to need a clear airway to do any good, and pinching the patient's nose closed will make your efforts more effective. Twelve to fifteen breaths per minute is a good rate to shoot for (have someone else time you, if possible), and skin color will be a good measure of how you're doing.

Shock

1. Send for help
2. Position head
   a) down if no head injury
   b) level to slightly elevated if head injury
3. Ensure airway
4. Control obvious bleeding
5. Keep patient warm
6. Attempt to improve circulation (see text)

Shock is essentially a depressed state affecting many vital organs, and caused by a relative decrease in blood supply to these organs. Symptoms include paleness or dusky skin color, cold or clammy perspiration, thirst, weakness, anxiety, nausea, and possibly vomiting.

In the visceral reaction (see above) fear causes the patient to "dump" blood into his deep visceral organs, thus depriving skin, head and muscle of their usual blood supply. This condition is temporary and will be relieved by soothing and calming measures.

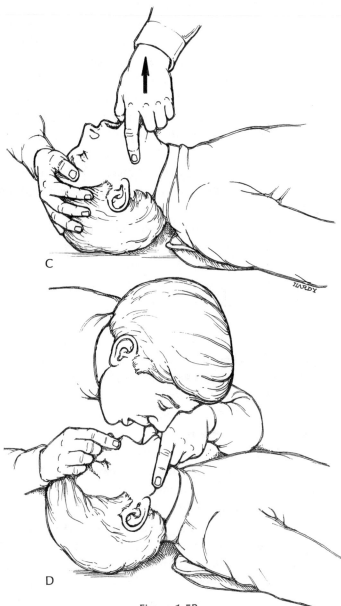

C

D

Figure 1-5B.

On the other hand, bleeding, either glaringly obvious or internal and sneaky, produces the same symptom complex. However, these symptoms will not respond until the patient gets competent *professional* medical care. This is what you can do until help arrives. (See Fig. 1-6)

Unless a head injury is suspected, the head-down position is best. With the patient lying supine, the legs should be slightly elevated so that the bottom half of the patient is higher than the top. Don't prop the buttocks as this will have a tendency to displace the abdominal contents up against the diaphragm and make breathing more difficult.

Sometimes the patient shows signs of shock while sitting, but it's inconvenient or impossible to lay him down. In this instance the head can be lowered between the knees, but the arms must be *down* so that the hands touch the floor. If the elbows are propped on the thighs, the head *cannot* get low enough.

The sitting, head-down position has another advantage, especially when used to treat the visceral reaction. The abdomen is compressed, forcing blood out of the viscera and back into the rest of the body.

There is one other relatively simple way one can improve circulation in a patient in shock. As a passenger on an airplane one time, I was called to see a man who was in obvious shock for unknown reasons. The stewardess had loosened his collar and belt and was getting out some oxygen. Why do people always loosen the belt? I can understand the collar (to ease breathing) but why the belt?

Utilizing principles I had learned as a flight surgeon, I remembered that compression suits were used to force blood from the abdomen up to the head in an effort to combat the effects of increased gravity. I stuffed two

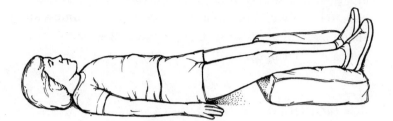

Shock positioning with no head injury

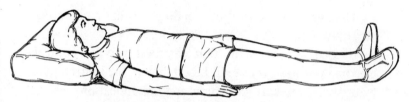

Positioning when head injury is present

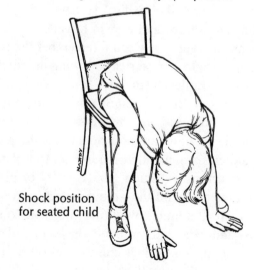

Shock position
for seated child

Figure 1-6.

folded copies of the *New York Times* under his belt and tightened it as snugly as he could tolerate; the color came back to his face and he felt a lot better. In shock, unless an abdominal injury is suspected, tighten the belt, don't loosen it. Your patient will thank you.

CONTROL OF BLEEDING

More Pressure—Fewer Points

The answer to control of bleeding is DIRECT PRESSURE ON THE WOUND!

It used to be taught that the best way to control bleeding was to slow arterial blood flow to the injured part by applying pressure to certain anatomic locations where arteries were most readily compressible. The only problem was that people were like medical students; they found anatomy difficult to learn and easy to forget!

Since in an emergency few could remember the correct pressure point, people then started following the teachings of the proverbial Little Dutch Boy. Where they saw the hole, they plugged it. But not wanting to put anything *into* the wound they plugged up the outside. And this has turned out to be the best and most reasonable thing to do.

Most children's wounds that require control of bleeding are on an arm or leg. Put a handkerchief or piece of cloth (clean preferably) on the wound and grasp it firmly. Hold it for 15 to 20 minutes, WITHOUT LOOKING TO SEE IF IT STOPPED, and you will probably have the bleeding stopped. If not, try another 20-minute period and then look again. This will control 95 percent of all bleeding wounds. (See Fig. 1-7)

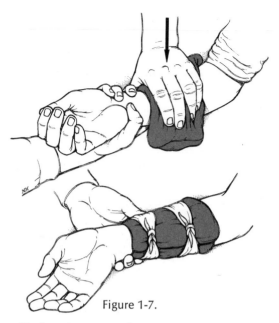

Figure 1-7.

If it still hasn't stopped, wrap it tightly, tie the wrapping in place and seek professional help. There may be an artery or arteriole (little artery) spurting, and you'll need medical help. If the wrapping controls the bleeding, (and it should), you don't have to pass any red lights to get to the doctor's office or emergency room.

Some children's wounds are not on an extremity, but regardless of where they are, direct pressure may be applied without damaging consequences. Some notable exceptions are the front of the neck and throat area, the eye, the genitalia in boys, and the abdomen if a deeper or more significant abdominal injury is suspected. (See "shock" above) These wounds will only tolerate *gentle* pressure which may not stop the bleeding, and professional medical help may have to be sought.

Since you can stop the bleeding in most of the wounds

you'll encounter, you now have time to examine the injury more carefully, cleanse it superficially for a better look if necessary, and make intelligent judgments about whether or not professional consultation is required. See Chapter 2.

OTHER CONSIDERATIONS

Immobilization—To Move or Not to Move

In twenty years of pediatric practice I have seen one spine injury in which movement of the patient was *contraindicated* until it could be done professionally. On the other hand, I've seen lots of patients left in snow, wet, blood, vomitus and many other undesirable situations for *fear* of moving him. Knowledge of a few facts in these instances would have made for better care.

Infants and toddlers aren't very fragile. As a matter of fact, they're pretty supple throughout and bend quite readily without breaking. However, they may not be able to tell you where they hurt, or what they can or cannot do with their arms and legs. (This would also be true of an unconscious patient.) A simple way to determine whether a small child or unconscious patient can be moved is to see if he has spontaneous movements of all four extremities.*

If the small child is moving all extremities but one, look to that extremity for an injury. If you find one (gross deformity, something out of joint, bruise or bleeding) that

---

* Spontaneous movement may be ascertained in the unconscious patient by pinching a finger or toe on each extremity. Depending on the depth of unconsciousness, most patients will try to withdraw the extremity when pain is produced.

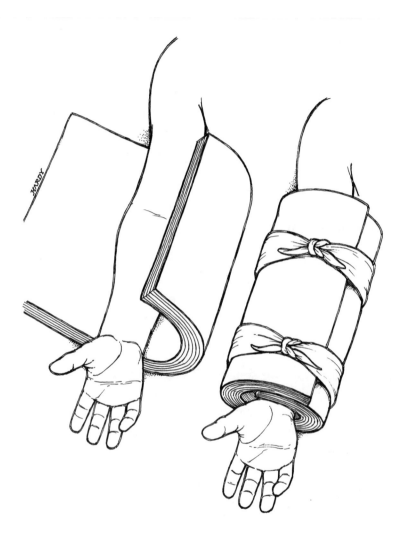

Figure 1-8.

extremity should be immobilized and then the child may be moved.

The immobilization of an extremity can be accomplished by any firm wrapping. A board, plank, pillow, rolled up newspaper, folded blanket or overcoat—almost anything wrapped around or placed under the patient's injured part will probably provide adequate immobilization temporarily and will allow you to make the patient more comfortable (Fig. 1-8). Move him if necessary and keep him warm. Standard first aid manuals may be consulted for more on this subject.

Do Not Move the Child if one of the following situations exists:

1. No extremity moves
2. Only one extremity moves
3. Both extremities on one side do not move (i.e., right arm and leg *or* left arm and leg
4. Neither leg moves

In the first three situations listed above, there's a good possibility that a spinal injury is present high in the neck. The fourth instance may involve a low back injury. All of these examples will require careful neurological evaluation and are best left to the professionals (See Fig. 1-9).

There are only two other possibilities. Contralateral limb disfunction (right arm and left leg, or vice versa) probably means that the injuries are limited to those extremities. (Immobilize the affected limbs and then the patient may be moved.)

Lack of function of both arms, with good leg usage, implies injuries of both arms. An example of this might be a child who falls and tries to break his fall with stretched

Figure 1-9. Move if:

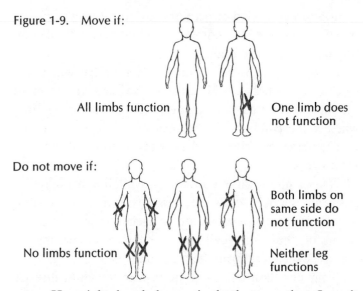

All limbs function

One limb does
not function

Do not move if:

Both limbs on
same side do
not function

No limbs function

Neither leg
functions

arms. He might break bones in both arms, but I can't think of a spinal injury that would affect both arms selectively and exclusively. Immobilize and move!

Determining the necessity for immobilization will be easier in an older child who is conscious and cooperative. He can tell you which limbs function and which do not. He can tell you where he hurts, and if you gently feel his spine, from neck to buttocks, he can tell you if he is acutely tender in a spot there. Absence of symptoms (what the patient tells you) and signs (what you find out by examining the patient) of a spinal injury will make you feel better about moving the patient.

Where to Get Help

I am basically rooted in the conviction that the best medical help available to your child will be provided by your family physician or pediatrician. And I firmly believe that the physician who knows your child best will take the best possible care of him.

So by all means call your doctor first. He will know whether or not the child needs to be seen, if the child should be referred immediately to another physician, whether the child should be seen in the office or at the local emergency room, and possibly if the child should have x rays made.

If your physician is not readily available, his office or answering service can usually direct your next move. You may be referred to a substitute physician or an emergency room, or they may call an ambulance or paramedic emergency team to bring help to you.

Your next best bet might be to take the child directly to the doctor's office or emergency room. That's all right, but I still urge you to call first or you might arrive only to find out the the doctor isn't in—or you're 99th on the list at the local emergency room.

Some of this confusion might be obviated if you asked your physician, during some non-emergency visit, exactly what you should do when you have an emergency. Facilities vary so widely from one community to another that the recommendations I have listed may not be appropriate in your situation, so find out how to get help *before* you need it!

The Tetanus Story

Most children have their basic immunizations against tetanus established early in childhood. Tetanus is included in the three DPT shots—diphtheria, pertussis (whooping cough), and tetanus—that they have early in their first year.

A booster is usually scheduled around 18 months and another pre-school (5 or 6 years). Between these immunizations (i.e., 6 months to 18 months, and 18 months to 5 years) they NEVER need boosters, regardless of what injuries they sustain.

After their pre-school booster, the recommendation for additional boosters is as follows;

1. routinely every 10 years
2. when injured
    a. no booster necessary if the child has had one in the last five years.
    b. booster if the wound is dirty or contaminated and the last booster occurred between 5-10 years ago.
    c. booster if the last one was over 10 years ago or the patient doesn't know.

Read this section carefully. We give far *fewer* boosters now than we did in the past.

2

Cuts and Lacerations—
Do They Need Stitches?

Cuts (smooth, clean slices through skin) and lacerations (jagged, rough tears of the skin) occur in a variety of sizes, shapes and locations. They usually heal, with or without help and with more or less scarring, if a reasonable amount of care and cleanliness is provided.

However, they will heal more quickly and with less scarring if the edges of the wound are brought together. How best to do this is the problem and an understanding of the properties of skin and how wound healing occurs will be helpful in solving it.

PROPERTIES OF SKIN THAT INFLUENCE HEALING

Mobility and Elasticity

Skin is both *mobile* and *elastic*. The mobility of skin is best demonstrated where it covers a joint. Consider the skin of your wrist. As the wrist is cocked up and down, the skin moves considerably to accommodate the swing of the hand.

Look at your wrist closely. It has furrows or ridges which run transversely across the wrist. These are called Langer's lines. (Fig. 2-1) Because of the mobility of the skin, when it is cut in the *same* direction as these lines, the wound edges are easy to pull together and less scarring is apt to occur.

On the other hand, when skin is cut perpendicular to Langer's lines, the *elasticity* of skin becomes more obvious because the wound edges *retract* and even the most finely incised line becomes a gaping wound. As you will see below, the direction of a skin cut as it relates to Langer's

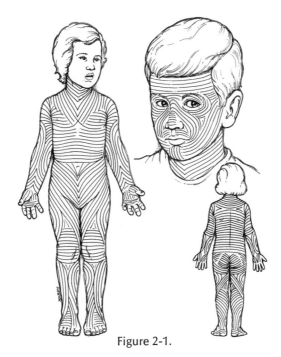

Figure 2-1.

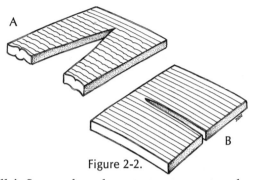

Figure 2-2.

lines will influence how best to treat a cut or laceration. (Fig. 2-2)

Wound Healing

Skin heals itself by filling its wounds with scar tissue. This process is accomplished from the depth of the wound up to the skin surface, just as you might fill in a deep rut in the driveway, from the bottom up. However, this is where the similarity ends.

The mobility and elasticity of skin allows us to move the edges of the wound closer together, so that there is less of a defect and therefore less tissue to be formed. Moving the skin together is easy; keeping it there while the wound heals is another story. (Fig. 2-3)

Skin Approximation (Bringing Wound Edges Together)

The two most common methods of keeping wound edges together are suturing (stitching) and bandaging (taping). From time to time, other methods have been

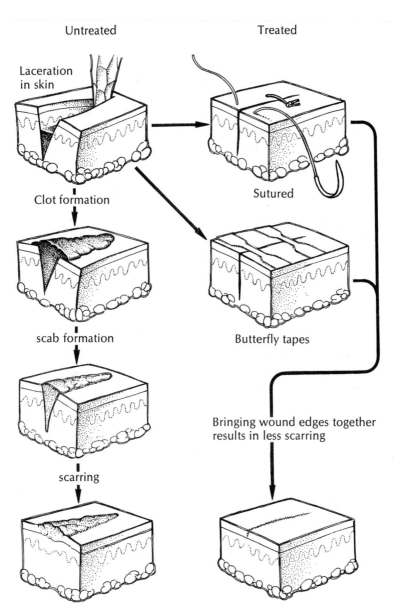

Untreated

Treated

Laceration in skin

Clot formation

Sutured

scab formation

Butterfly tapes

Bringing wound edges together results in less scarring

scarring

Figure 2-3.

tried (staples, clips, etc.) but they have never found favor in this country.

Suturing requires professional care. It is necessary to sterilize the wound, use sterile needles, thread and instruments, and know what one is doing. This type of closure provides the best cosmetic result, with the least amount of scarring and the shortest healing time. But all wounds do not *need* to be sutured. As a matter of fact, I believe that some wounds should *not* be stitched.

The decision to sew or not to sew should be made after consideration of many factors. Let us consider these factors.

Size and Shape of the Wound

Most wounds are linear—that is, they are longer than they are wide. Although the skin is cut, there usually is no significant loss of flesh—all of the cloth is there, it just needs repairing. When a wound is straight and clean it may very well be a candidate for bandages rather than sutures.

Generally speaking, the longer the wound, the more likely it will need stitches. Again, where to draw the line may be difficult. A half-inch *gaping* wound of the face should be stitched, whereas a two-inch wound of the lower abdomen might be very amenable to taping.

Wounds that are jagged, ugly, irregular or have destroyed and macerated flesh should probably have competent professional care. They will usually need to be revised (have some plastic surgery) to improve their appearance and make wound-edge approximation easier before they are closed. (Fig. 2-4)

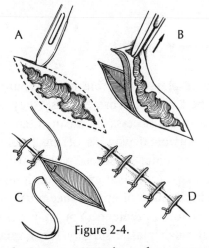

Figure 2-4.

Some wounds are cut or torn in such a way as to raise a flap of skin, almost completely separate from the body, save for a small bridge of tissue. If the blood supply to the flap has been seriously compromised, the flap may turn very dark, or even black. The best treatment for this type of wound is to have professional care. If the flap is hopelessly devoid of blood supply, it should be removed and the wound revised in such a way as to allow skin closure. If not, sutures will usually be required to give the flap the best possible chance of healing.

Orientation to Langer's Lines

As mentioned earlier, linear wounds that run in the same direction as Langer's lines will close more readily than those that run across the lines. This will be obvious because of the degree of gaping seen. Most wounds that gape considerably require sutures, although again, other factors need to be considered.

Location of the Wound

Cosmetics plays a big role here. Wounds of the face want the best possible care because they are so visible. Still, this does not necessarily mean stitches in all cases. I have seen horizontal wounds of the forehead heal perfectly well in older children with nary a scar when appropriate tape is applied and left on long enough.

The consideration of appearance must weigh future as well as present requirements. You may not want to put a little girl through plastic surgery for a small but jagged laceration of the breast, but in 20 years she might wish you had.

Some wounds produce wide scars regardless of how well you treat them. Elbows and knees are notorious for this. The mobility of the joint, and therefore the skin covering it, always seems to stretch and widen the scar. Therefore the decision to sew in these areas should probably be governed more by function than by cosmetics.

Some wounds may be in areas with a notoriously poor blood supply. A good example is the shin, where the skin lies directly on top of bone and there is no subcutaneous tissue to supply nutrient blood to the skin. Wounds here heal with some difficulty and may need all the help they can get. Probably a case for stitches.

Function of the Underlying Part

Knee and elbow wounds discussed above are good examples of this consideration. An inactive child whose limb can be partially immobilized by a thick bandage for a week will probably heal perfectly well with tape. (The same is true, for instance, of knuckles, shoulder and hip.) However, wounds in these same locations had best be sewn if the child cannot be kept relatively inactive. (If the knee laceration of a runner is well sewn, he can be in the track meet—stitches still in—in a day or so.)

An untrained toddler who sits on a scissors and sustains a laceration of the buttock had best be well cleansed and stitched quickly. The wound will heal in the shortest possible time, making less likely an infection from soiled diapers.

A boy may have to shave over a lumpy, uneven scar on his chin for the rest of his life, even though he was beardless when he cut himself. Better to get it sutured.

Sex of the Patient

A girl's neck, shoulders, arms, and legs are frequently exposed, and cuts on these parts deserve the most careful treatment.

Scars on boys are still more readily accepted, so in borderline cases you might decide to bandage rather than stitch.

Age of the Patient

Most toddlers will have to be held or tied down before they can have sutures placed. This is a real trauma and can set back a good doctor-patient relationship for months or even years. Therefore, whenever possible, tape rather than sutures should be used.

Unfortunately this may *not* be possible for a variety of reasons. For one, a toddler cannot be trusted to leave the bandage in place. For another, cosmetic considerations may make stitches mandatory. Frequently, the decision to tape or stitch is a real conundrum. I guess the best way to sum it up would be to say that if there is no overriding need to suture, and if the difference between the width of the scars is only 1 to 3 millimeters (less than ⅛ inch), I'd opt for the tape and settle for the slightly larger scar.

Season of the Year

Wounds that are taped need to be kept dry for at least three to five days. That means no swimming. Perspiration will also loosen tape. With stitches in an uncomplicated wound, a child can swim in 36 to 48 hours (with the stitches still in. Obviously the dressing will have to be changed).

Similarly, it's tough to tell an older child he can't go skiing during his Christmas vacation just because his wound might open. It's easier to sew the wound closed in the first place, apply a protective dressing and send him to the slopes.

Cleanliness of the Wound

Some wounds should never be closed. Human bites have a very high incidence of infection (the mouth has been likened to a sewer) and if cosmetics are not important, are best left open to heal.*

If the bite is in a bad location cosmetically, a surgeon will frequently close the wound after Herculean efforts at sterilization and put the child on prophylactic antibiotics.

Knee lacerations with ground-in dirt are frequently left to heal without wound closure because of the likelihood of infection caused by multiple foreign bodies. Similarly, cuts in the diaper area, very close to the anus, may be left open. If the child has chronic diarrhea, the surgeon may not wish to risk an infection deep in the closed wound.

Excessive Bleeding

Many wounds need to have stitches to stop bleeding. As an example, lacerations of the scalp (which has a very rich blood supply) frequently need to be sutured closed for this reason. Tape alone won't stop the bleeding.

Similarly, if a small artery or arteriole is cut, one sees blood being spurted out. The frequency of the spurts matches pulse rate, and the blood will always be more scarlet in color. Stitches will almost invariably be required in these cases.

Psychological and Financial Considerations

I have alluded previously to the psychological trauma to the toddler who needs to be forcibly held down to have

---

* Foreign material or bacteria may be injected into the wound at the time of injury and be very difficult to cleanse properly. If the wound is closed, an incubator effect is created which propagates bacterial growth.

a wound properly sutured. In certain situations this might also be true of an older child.

One might ask why a child shouldn't be put to sleep to have a wound properly treated. If you stop and consider that there is risk associated with any type of general anesthesia, the answer will be obvious. Unless a wound is quite extensive, the potential for psychological trauma probably doesn't justify the anesthetic risk, however small.

It is also necessary to consider the question of finances. Taping at home is free. Suturing is surgery, and surgeons (or physicians who do surgery) are expensive. More than one visit is usually involved, and fees mount up. Even if insurance makes the cost factor seem inconsequential, we must one day face up to the fact that premiums rise, and we'll all pay sooner or later.

Therefore, although I certainly don't advocate saving money at the expense of adequate treatment, if the difference in the end result will be negligible, those dollars are just as useful in your pocket as they are in the doctor's.

MAKING THE JUDGMENT

Taking into account as many of the above factors as possible, one must decide whether the child is to be treated at home (with bandaging) or at a medical facility (with stitching). This may not be easy, but here are some guidelines.

First, remember that you can change your mind. If you try to tape the wound and are not happy with the way the wound comes together, you can always take the child to the doctor.

Second, even after healing, an unsatisfactory cosmetic

result can usually be surgically revised. Although it is certainly true that in some situations the first attempt is the one most likely to achieve the best result, this is not usually true with a simple, relatively minor wound.

If, on balance, you can't decide which type of treatment might be best, by all means try to tape the wound shut yourself. (See p. 58 for step-by-step instructions.)

One warning! Most physicians will not close a wound that has been open longer than six hours. The danger of infection is too great. So if you're not happy with your result, don't wait until "tomorrow" to ask the physician to fix it.

Finally, in all your deliberations, keep the welfare of the total child in mind, not just the wound, and remember that the primary concern is the end result, not just the difficulty, discomfort or unhappiness of the immediate situation.

TREATMENT OF OPEN WOUNDS AT HOME

This section appears in check-list form for purposes of ready reference in an emergency. Like most of this book, it should be read first in a non-emergency situation to familiarize yourself with general content and location of detail. It will then be easier to use as specific situations arise.

1. Your Immediate Response

The following things should be done first, and virtually simultaneously:

    a. *Comfort the child.* Hold him or her and soothe, comfort and reassure. (Fig. 2-5)

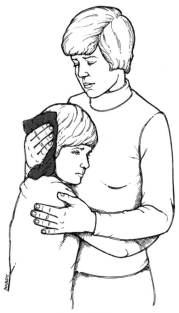

Figure 2-5.

b. *Control bleeding with direct pressure.* Use almost any reasonably clean piece of cloth, paper or even your bare hand.

c. *Enlist the aid of some other adult,* older child in the home or a neighbor.

2. Think: Your Second Response

Make a *preliminary* judgment about how care is to be accomplished. Either:

a. *This needs professional care.* If so, immobilize as

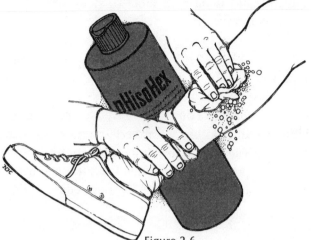

Figure 2-6.

necessary, control bleeding and make arrangements to transport. If time permits, look up the date of the child's last tetanus booster, make arrangements for the care of the other children, and leave a message for your spouse—he or she will be frantic.

or   b. *Can handle this one myself.* (Skip to #3)

or   c. *Don't know yet!* Can't make the judgment as yet—there's still too much bleeding. I don't have enough light, can't quiet the child. I could probably do it if I had some help, etc., etc. Will continue to treat and reserve judgment for a few minutes.

3. Check List for Home Treatment

Bleeding has stopped; child is quiet; neighbor or older child is helping; bandage and cleaning materials at hand, good light, child is on bed, table or floor where I have plenty of room to work.

4. Exposure

Expose wound. You may have to remove some clothing. (Cutting clothing off is very dramatic but seldom necessary.) It can usually be slipped off gently, but cut if you must. Exposure may also involve cutting some hair, even some shaving to expose wound edges. (This is mandatory in scalp wounds.)

5. Cleansing

Cleanse wound. Soap—any kind is good. Liquid soap containing hexachlorophene (pHisoHex) is best. Get a prescription from your doctor now so you will have it on hand. It should be used with plenty of warm water, and gauze pads, wash cloth or similar. Don't use absorbent cotton or paper tissues—they shred and may leave remnants in the wound. (Fig. 2-6) P.S.—Don't be afraid of hexachlorophene. The notoriety of this substance comes only from whole-body scrubs of newborn infants over several days. Its use in the cleansing of wound infections is perfectly safe and proper.

Gentle scrubbing with pHisoHex is a better cleansing method than patting with antiseptic solutions. Alcohol burns like blazes, iodine destroys tissue; Zephiran hydrochloride frequently loses potency and becomes unsterile; patent first aid creams are almost worthless, Mercurochrome (merbromin) colors the wound red, so you

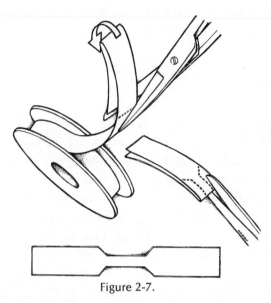

Figure 2-7.

have a hard time later deciding whether the wound is reddening because of infection.

And don't be afraid to re-start bleeding. A little more bleeding is also cleansing, and if you've stopped the bleeding once you can do it again!

6. Preparing for Tape

To prepare the wound for better adhesive adherence, the edges should be thoroughly dried and hair should be removed. Alcohol and acetone (the main ingredient in nail polish remover)—applied to skin around the wound—are good drying agents. A compound called tincture of benzoin may be applied around the wound to increase the "stickiness" of the surface.

CAUTION—Don't "blow" any of these surfaces dry.

You're blowing mouth bacteria into the wound. Rather, fan them dry before applying adhesive.

7. Taping

You're now ready to tape the wound edges together. Butterfly bandages contain two relatively large surfaces for each side of the wound and a thin bridge of non-adhesive cloth to bridge or cross the wound. They are available commercially from Johnson and Johnson in three sizes.

They may also be fashioned from ordinary adhesive tape by doing simple cutting and folding. Their size should match the length of the wound. (See Fig. 2-7)

A technique that works well for me is to apply a large butterfly temporarily to the center of the wound as a holding device. This should have a long, narrow bridge with the large adhesive ends back and away from the wound. After any oozing of blood is cleansed away, multiple small butterflies may be applied on either side of the temporary central one. (Fig. 2-8)

8. More Taping

The "holding" butterfly may now be removed, but BE CAREFUL! Its edges should be lifted on the same side of both flaps and it should gently be pulled off so that the force is exerted in the *same* direction as the long axis of the wound! (See Fig. 2-9) Thus, you will not be exerting any pressure against the holding action of the other butterflies, and there will be less tendency to separate the wound edges.

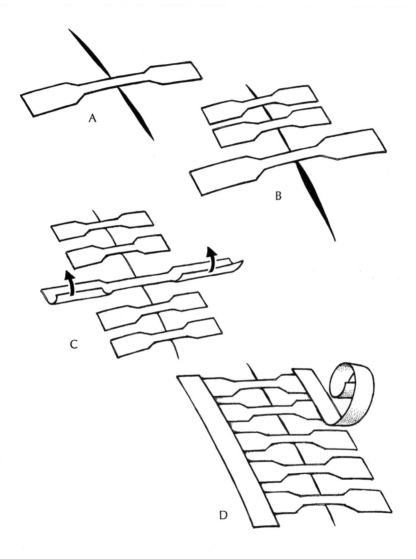

Figure 2-8.

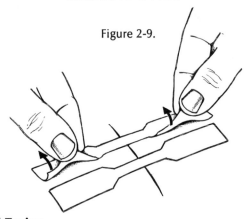

Figure 2-9.

9. Final Taping

More small butterflies may now be applied, if necessary, to the center of the wound. Further, a strip of adhesive may be applied to cross all the flaps on either side of the wound, lending strength and increasing the adherent adhesive surface area.

A large bandage may now be applied to cover the whole construction. Take care not to allow the adhesive of the outer dressing to touch the adhesive of any of the butterfly construction. (The outer dressing may have to be changed, but the butterflies had best be left alone for at least a week.)

10. Check for Infection

The outer dressing should be changed in 24 to 48 hours to check for infection. Redness, heat, swelling and tenderness are the cardinal signs. Pus may be present. If infection is suspected, *all* the tape should be removed and the wound split open. (This will be easier than it sounds.)

It should be washed with pHisoHex as described above and a series of warm soaks (20 to 30 minutes three to four times a day in a basin with a quart of warm water and a tablespoon of Epsom salts) begun. An antibiotic ointment (Bacitracin, Neopolycin, or Neosporin) may be applied after soaking and before rebandaging. If fever is present, a physician should be consulted. Without fever, the soaks should be continued until the wound closes by itself (10 to 14 days) and there is no further evidence of drainage when the bandage is removed.

If in trying to remove the bandage you find that it sticks to the wound, it may be soaked off, or soaked with ordinary drug store hydrogen peroxide which will "bubble" it off. At the next dressing be sure to use a liberal quantity of antibiotic ointment to keep the dressing lubricated. It won't stick to the wound again.

11. Duration of Treatment

If no infection is found after the first dressing, there is a reasonable degree of assurance that the wound will heal nicely. The butterflies should be left on for at least five to seven days; in areas of great elasticity (knees and elbows) or increased exposure to trauma (hands, feet, etc.), try to leave them on for 10 to 14 days after the injury occurred.

A wound does not achieve its greatest tensile strength for 14 days—so even after the butterflies come off, maintain a dressing until the wound is two weeks old. During this time the outer dressing may be changed as often as necessary (as determined by its appearance) but at least every two to three days to check on the progress of healing.

If butterfly tapes are to remain firmly in place the wound must be kept dry! This is a definite disadvantage of this method, but there's *no way* that tape is going to hold if it gets wet. You're just going to have to bathe around the bandage, and probably the patient will exhibit some visible dirt. But the end result will be worth it, and you can take justifiable pride in your work.

FISHHOOKS—A SPECIAL SITUATION

The fishhook caught in human skin is really a special kind of cut/laceration situation. This deserves mention here because it is so common an occurrence in children of all ages.

Look at the anatomy of a fishhook! One or more *barbed* heads, and an eyelet tail. It is designed so that once flesh is impaled on it, it *won't pull out!* So don't try unless you can *see* the barb! (Fig. 2-10)

If the barb is *very* superficial and you can envision a *very short* path for it to be *pushed* through and out, you may try this. You'll need a cooperative child and some

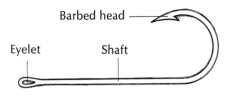

Figure 2-10

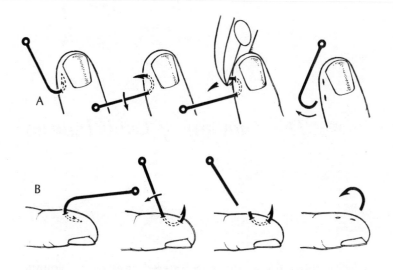

Figure 2-11.

snips to cut the barb of the hook, so you can slide the hook gently out of the entry hold. (Fig. 2-11)

Following this, remember that you're dealing with a potentially infected puncture wound. Clean the area thoroughly, apply antiseptic and start warm soaking 20 minutes, three to four times per day. Tetanus boosters should be checked, and watch for infection (increased tenderness, redness, swelling, heat, streaks on the adjacent areas, or pus).

But really—the pro can do this job so much better, quicker, easier and relatively painlessly. A drop of locally infiltrated anesthetic and a sharp sterile scalpel makes all the difference in the world. So if you're squeamish, the child is uncooperative or the hook is deeply set, get help!

And remember to check on tetanus!

3

The Anatomy of Limb Injuries

The most frequently encountered injuries in youngsters occur to their limbs. The developing child, exploding with curiosity, uses his arms, hands and fingers to explore the environment; he uses his legs to get him there. As he comes into contact with previously unknown hazards, he sometimes gets injured.

When a child hurts himself, he doesn't tell a parent he has a "fracture of the second phalangeal bone of the fourth digit of his right hand." He comes into the house and says "Mommie, I hurt my finger!" To deal with the problem the parent must first know what precisely is wrong with the finger.

Let us then learn how to diagnose injuries of the extremities. First we need to know a little anatomy, so that we can figure out which structures may be injured. Then we can take up the types of injuries that occur to these structures. Finally, we will consider the injuries which

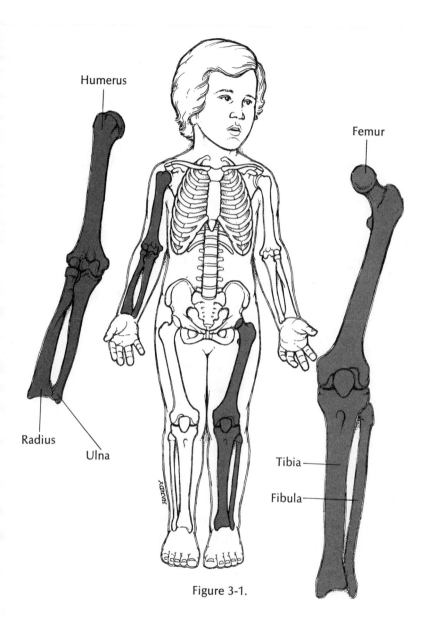

Figure 3-1.

commonly occur to children in varying locations, and what to do about them.

ANATOMY OF THE LIMBS

Bones

The structural framework on which limbs are built. The major long bones of the upper and lower extremity are shown in Fig. 3-1.

Joints

The "hinges" or points of articulation between bones that move. Joints limit the type of motion that may occur between bones to specific planes or directions. The shoulder and hip are examples of "ball and socket" joints that allow a relatively great range of motion in many directions. The elbow and knee are hinge-type joints which allow movement in only one plane or direction. (Fig. 3-2)

Ligaments

Fibrous bands of very strong connective tissue that surround and frequently enclose joints. They must be strong enough to keep the bones in place, yet flexible enough to allow them to move in controlled directions. (Fig. 3-3)

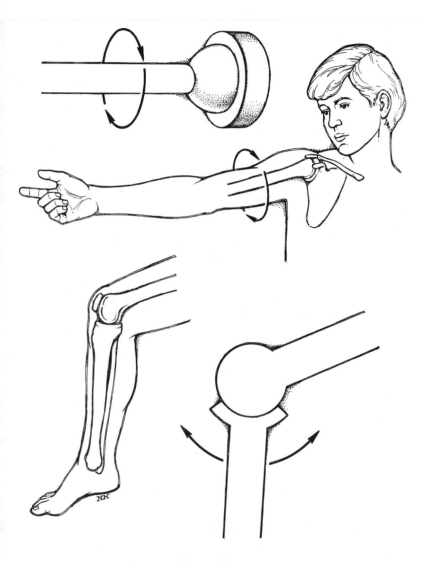

Figure 3-2.

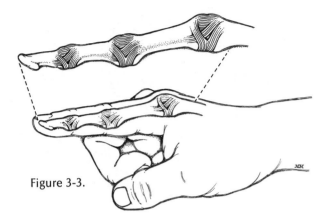

Figure 3-3.

Muscles

Provide the power to move bones and therefore limbs. They may be likened to springs that expand or contract on demand, thus lengthening or shortening the distance between bones by creating motion at the joint. (Fig. 3-4)

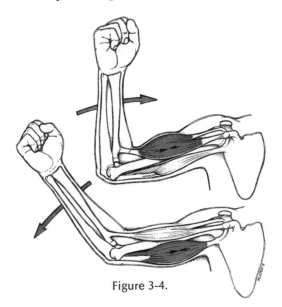

Figure 3-4.

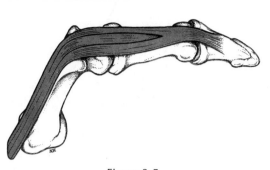

Figure 3-5.

Tendons

Thick, white, ropelike structures that blend into muscles at one end and attach to bone at the other. Tendons usually cross joints, thus enabling muscles to move one bone relative to another, at the joint. (Fig. 3-5)

Cartilage

Firm, but not completely rigid tissue—the stuff that bones are made of, before they are infiltrated with hard calcium salts. Most cartilage in kids gets calcified eventually. Some does not.

The knee (Fig. 3-6) is an example of an area in which cartilage provides a smooth, relatively friction-free surface where one bone can move against another without creating undue trauma. This action may be likened to that of ball bearings.

Figure 3-6.

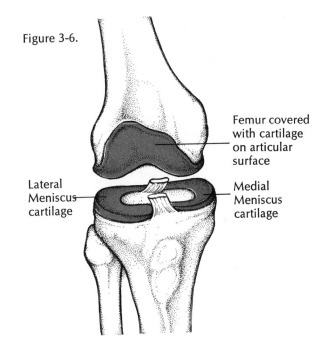

Femur covered
with cartilage
on articular
surface

Lateral
Meniscus
cartilage

Medial
Meniscus
cartilage

Obviously this is a simplification of all the anatomical structures that occur in extremities, but for our purposes it will suffice. Let us now consider how these structures become injured, and the types of injuries that occur to them.

TYPES OF ANATOMICAL INJURIES

Contusions

Minor injuries to any part of the body, in which the skin and underlying soft tissues are bruised. They usually result from sharp blows and will cause discoloration (black-and-blue mark), minor swelling and tenderness.

Function (movement) is never lost, although it may be painful.

Abrasions

Scrapes of the skin surface, usually caused by a glancing blow and resulting in the shearing off of the outermost layer of skin. There may be some minor oozing of body tissues, or bleeding, and a good bit of pain as many tiny superficial pain fibers are laid bare and injured.

Strains

Injuries to muscles, and/or their attached tendons. They occur as the result of a stretching or pulling injury. The anatomy remains mostly intact, but there may be some minute, even microscopic, tearing of muscle bands or tendon fibers. This may be quite tender and painful. An example of this type of injury is the so-called "charley horse" which occurs most frequently in the calf or thigh muscles of the leg.

Sprains

Injuries in which ligaments are usually torn in or around the joint. The degree of severity of sprains is so variable that treatment may range from "none necessary" to immobilization with a plaster cast for three to six weeks. The ankle sprain is a typical example of this injury. (Fig. 3-7)

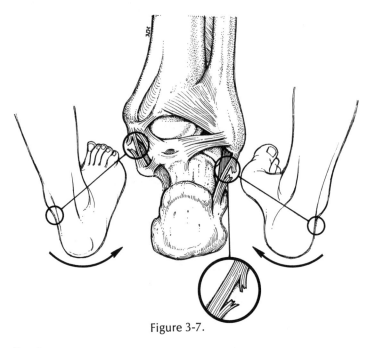

Figure 3-7.

Fractures

Broken bones. Let us set to rest the myth that there is any difference between a fracture and a broken bone. There is not. There are many types of fractures, and different ways to describe them. A brief summary which is illustrated by Fig. 3-8, will be helpful at this point.

SIMPLE FRACTURE (non-displaced). The bone is broken, with the ends slightly separated but in good alignment. No "setting" or manipulation is required, just immobilization.

DISPLACED FRACTURE. The two bone segments are in poor position. They may lie at an angle, or with the broken ends overriding. Setting or manipulation is required to straighten them before immobilization.

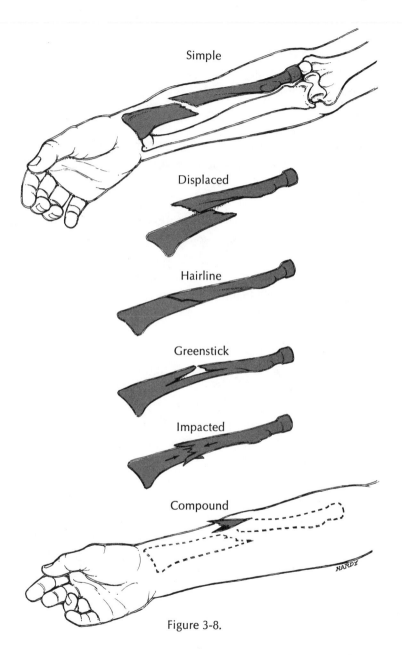

Simple

Displaced

Hairline

Greenstick

Impacted

Compound

Figure 3-8.

HAIRLINE FRACTURE. The bone is cracked, like a piece of porcelain or the crack in a wall or ceiling. This fracture may not be evident at the time of injury, *even by x ray,* but might become more obvious if the film is taken 7 to 10 days after the injury, when the repair process points to the fine crack in the bone. No setting required. Immobilization still necessary.

GREENSTICK FRACTURE. Only a portion of the shaft of the bone is broken. Imagine trying to break a "green" or live branch of a tree. Even though you may bend it double, only part of the limb breaks; part remains intact. Very common in children. Immobilization by a physician is necessary. He will also decide whether setting is necessary.

IMPACTED FRACTURE. The fragmented ends of the bone are jammed together, almost as if the injury broke the bone and tried to fix it at the same time. Depending on position, this fracture may or may not require manipulation. But immobilization will be necessary.

COMPOUND FRACTURE. The fragmented end of bone is associated with a laceration of the skin and may *protrude* (or have protruded at the moment of injury) through the skin. A very severe injury requiring immediate professional care. Cleanliness as a first aid measure (or rather protection against further contamination and infection) is vital.

There are several other types of anatomical injury; we will touch on them briefly as the need arises. For our general purpose, however, contusions, abrasions, strains, sprains, and fractures are the ones most commonly encountered by children. They will occupy most of our attention.

4

Injuries to the Upper Limb

When a child injures part of the upper extremity it may be difficult to tell which portion has been injured. This is especially true if the child is very young, very upset or crying so much that he won't respond to your queries. The only obvious sign may be that he won't use the arm.

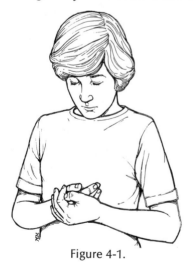

Figure 4-1.

The hand may be an exception. If the hand or fingers are injured, the child will hold the hand up and the injury to the hand or fingers will probably be obvious. But if the injury is above the hand, the whole arm will probably be immobile. (Fig. 4-1)

One then needs to examine the whole arm. This should include the shoulder and the area between the shoulder and the neck in front of and above the chest; fracture of the clavicle occurs here.

FRACTURE OF THE CLAVICLE

One of the bones most often broken in early childhood, the clavicle or collar bone may be fractured by a direct blow along its shaft, or more commonly by falling forward on the rigid outstretched arm. Force is transmitted up the arm and impacts on one of the curves of the clavicle. This bone is rigidly attached to the sternum and thus the chest wall. (Fig. 4-2)

Because movement of any part of the arm is transmitted to the clavicle, pain occurs at the fracture site, and thus the arm is held limply. Gentle touching of the arm should begin at the clavicle. The fracture site is quite tender; the youngster will immediately identify this as the source of his pain. Sometimes the fracture is evident merely by looking at it, since the bone is directly beneath the skin, with no intervening muscle mass to hide the injury. One is likely to see a *bump* or mass, corresponding to the point of tenderness.

Frequently the injury, when first called to the attention of a parent, is a day or two old. It seems strange that a bone can be broken without great discomfort, but some-

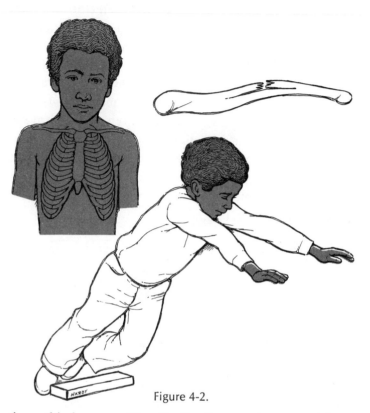

Figure 4-2.

times this happens. Usually the fracture is greenstick, or hairline, or impacted in such a way that no motion is allowed. With minimal motion at the fracture site, there may be minimal discomfort. The parent usually feels guilty that an injury of this magnitude went unnoticed.

Sometimes attention is called to the bump by an overlying area of discoloration *(ecchymosis* or black and blue). The broken bone has bled directly beneath the skin and discoloration shows through.

In summary, the diagnosis of a fractured clavicle is made by knowing how the injury was sustained, by looking for immobility, discoloration and/or a bump along the shaft of the bone that is sensitive when touched.

Treatment should be undertaken by the physician, who may want to confirm the evidence (x ray) and who will best know how to treat the particular type of fracture incurred. In most instances a simple method is used to immobilize *both* shoulders. Plaster is rarely used any more. A figure-eight bandage, pulling both shoulders back and crossing behind and between the shoulder blades is usually adequate. Commercial clavicle splints or shoulder braces are available. They are easy to apply and more comfortable to wear. (Fig. 4-3)

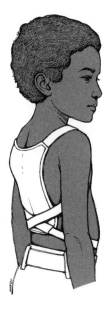

Figure 4-3.

The prognosis for healing a broken collarbone in the young child is excellent. Over the course of three weeks following the injury the previously noted bump will become larger, firmer and less tender. At the end of that time the fracture may be said to be functionally healed, and the immobilizing appliance may be removed. In the following months the bump (actually it's called a *callus*) will diminish in size, leaving *no* evidence of previous fracture. (Fig. 4-4)

One warning: In older children, especially pubertal and post-pubertal girls, great care must be taken in

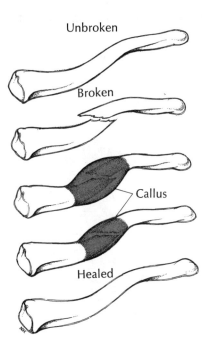

Figure 4-4.

aligning the fractured bone ends. Otherwise deformity may occur which is less than attractive when the shoulders are bare.

Other Shoulder Injuries

Rare in younger children; for purposes of this discussion may be discounted. Most impact and wrenching injuries result in soreness and discomfort and get better in a few days. Severe injuries: those that result in obvious deformity, and those in which very severe pain and limitation of motion are paramount symptoms, should be immobilized (Fig. 4-5) and brought to the physician. Fractures and severely torn ligaments occasionally occur and need professional help.

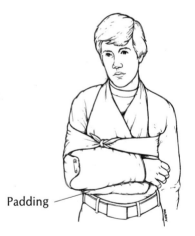

Padding

Figure 4-5.

The Upper Arm

May be broken, but this too is rare in childhood. Once again, deformity, limitation of motion and very severe pain, usually associated with swelling, are your best clues. If these symptoms and signs are present, the child should be immobilized very *carefully* (sling and swathe again) and brought to the physician. There is a real danger here of injury to blood vessels and nerves by the fragmented bone ends. Most often, however, a blow to the upper arm usually results in a "charley horse" (bruise) of the biceps or triceps muscle and will heal itself.

PULLED ELBOW—SUBLUXATION OF THE RADIAL HEAD

One injury common to toddlers, and most often inadvertently caused by an adult, is the subluxed radial head or pulled elbow. This also may be the perfect example of how a competent parent or adult can fix a child's injury, simply and easily, with a little knowledge.

Picture this: An adult and a child are walking along, usually in a hurry, the adult holding the child's hand. Stepping off a curb, the toddler trips. Instinctively the adult pulls up sharply on the child's hand in an attempt to keep the child on his feet. The elbow snaps, and the toddler cries out in pain. (Fig. 4-6)

Immediately it is evident that the child does not want to use the arm. Frequently he will hold his sore arm by the wrist or forearm with his good hand in a simple attempt at natural immobilization. And he will cry. (Fig. 4-7)

Perhaps when one encounters this situation for the first time, it might be best to let a physician handle it. But watch him very carefully, because this injury tends to recur, and if it happens again, you may want to treat it yourself.

The first step will be to quiet the the child and obtain his cooperation. This is necessary because you have to judge his reaction to the diagnostic maneuvers which will help you pinpoint the problem. Next, simple touching of the clavicle area, shoulder, upper arm (SKIP THE ELBOW for now), wrist, lower forearm and hand will point to the area of maximum discomfort.

Having ascertained that the problem is around the elbow and with the knowledge that the child has pulled it before, inspect the elbow carefully. If there are no gross deformities, it is reasonably safe to touch the area gently. Note that the elbow is partly bent and that the hand is

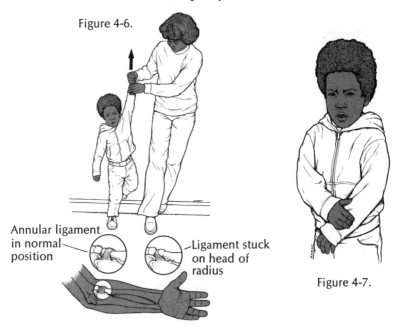

Figure 4-6.

Annular ligament in normal position

Ligament stuck on head of radius

Figure 4-7.

turned over, palm side down. Tenderness will be noted in the bend of the elbow when one touches this area gently.

When you've satisfied yourself that there are no *other* injuries of the arm and that the problem seems to center around the elbow, which is *not* grossly deformed, you are ready to relocate the radial head. Grasp the patient's wrist gently but firmly—your left to the patient's left or right to right. (Fig. 4-8) Lay the thumb of your other hand across the bend of his injured elbow, and grasp the back of the elbow firmly with your other fingers. Now, while exerting pressure with your thumb, straighten his elbow and rotate his wrist outward so that the palm is up, rather than down.

As you do this, you should feel a palpable and almost audible "click" as if something had "snapped" into place. There may be an immediate cry of pain from the patient but if you've been successful and heard or felt the click, you will note that when the youngster is again quieted down, he can be persuaded to move his arm and elbow without pain.

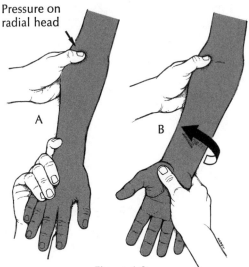

Pressure on radial head

A

B

Figure 4-8.

His motions will be gingerly and hesitant at first, but if you pass a small object back and forth between the two of you, alternating good and bad arms, you will note that he begins to use the arm in a way that he wouldn't before your manipulation. It may still be tender, and have some limitation of motion, but the improvement should be very obvious. A sling applied for 24 hours, or at least until bedtime that night, may be all you need to complete the treatment. If you try to apply the sling next day to the patient who's been cured, he probably won't tolerate it because he doesn't need it.

On the other hand, if your manipulation has *not* been obviously successful, you should seek professional help without delay, as a fracture or more serious dislocation are possibilities, and x rays and further professional examination and treatment are necessary.

In subluxation, the sooner the treatment after the injury the more quickly will the patient recover and the more dramatic will be the results of your successful manipulation. If the patient has been injured for some time before manipulation, the results may not be as dramatic, and the elbow may remain sore (even though it's been fixed) for 24 to 72 hours. This factor should enter into your decision to treat and your evaluation of the results of manipulation. (You may not want to treat it if the injury has been present for a day or so.)

FRACTURE OF THE FOREARM

Another fairly common injury of childhood is fracture of one or both bones of the forearm. The injury usually occurs from falling on one or both outstretched hands (similar to the injury that produces a fractured clavicle), and the break occurs in the forearm that bears the brunt of the fall. Most often the fracture is distal, or down at the end of the forearm near the wrist, and is frequently confused with a wrist injury.

The severity of this injury is variable. The angle between hand and forearm may create a deformity which is so obvious that diagnosis of fracture is readily evident (the so-called "silver fork" deformity of *Colle's fracture*). (Fig. 4-9) In this situation the whole forearm *and hand* is splinted on a flat board, and you're off to the doctor.

An impacted fracture, however, may show little or no deformity and swelling; only the persistence of pain and tenderness for a day or two may make you realize that this may be an injury that requires some professional care.

Consequently, *any injury of the forearm and/or wrist that shows deformity, swelling or persistent pain and/or*

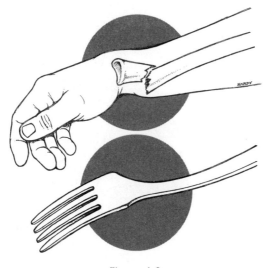

Figure 4-9.

tenderness should be seen professionally. X rays will almost certainly be required; many of these injuries will need further treatment.

INJURIES TO THE WRIST

The wrist, one of the most complex joints of the body, articulates two bones of the forearm with nine tiny bones. These are in turn connected to the five metacarpal bones of the hand. Numerous ligaments and tendons also go through the wrist, connecting muscles of the forearm which supply much of the motor power to the hand and fingers. (Fig. 4-10)

Although most of the injuries of the wrist involve minor sprains and tendon stretching, occasionally one finds a fracture of one of the tiny wrist bones or of the

Figure 4-10.

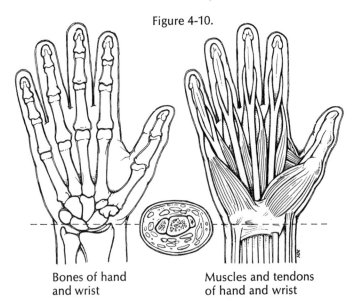

Bones of hand
and wrist

Muscles and tendons
of hand and wrist

ends of either the bones of the forearm or the metacarpals. These fractures are not usually displaced; little deformity or swelling is present. Motion at the wrist is not usually completely lost, although it may be diminished or painful.

Often when one x-rays the wrist right after an injury, a thin hairline fracture is not apparent, because its x-ray image is too fine, or because the bones overlay each other (the image is only two-dimensional). Fine detail may be difficult to pick up. Therefore in a child whose debility from a wrist injury is *not* severe, a prudent course might be to delay x-raying for a week or ten days. Then the process of repair may be easier to see on the x-ray film than the original fracture line. This is because the first stage of repair involves some dissolution of bone at the fracture site before new bone is laid down. Thus a film taken later will frequently show an aspect of *the* fracture—or even a second fracture—that may not have been picked up on a film done at the time of injury. And you will feel better for having checked.

In summary, then, injuries of the wrist may be difficult to diagnose because of the complex anatomy involved. The general treatments of "ice early, heat later," immobilization (any surgical supply house and many drug stores carry a variety of wrist-support and splint devices), and aspirin for pain are indicated. Depending upon the degree of disability, x-ray examination may be deferred for 7 to 10 days in the hope that a fracture, if present, may be more readily apparent.

Lacerations of the Wrist

One final word on the wrist: cuts on or near the wrist deserve special mention because of the number and complexity of nerves, ligaments, tendons and blood vessels which course through this narrow corridor. (See again Fig. 4-10)

It is therefore extremely important to test *every* function of the *hand* and *each finger.* Can a fist be made? Can the hand be cocked *up and down* on the wrist? Does each finger *flex* and *extend?* Can the fingers spread apart and close together so that they touch each other in the open palm or extended position?

Testing for *all* these functions is *mandatory* before one may assume that a wrist laceration is superficial and can be treated simply!

THE HAND

The bones of the hand, or metacarpals, break from time to time, but not often. The injury usually comes as the result of an improperly closed fist smashing against a hard object. (If your child must fight, teach him to close his fist tightly!) Since the hand bones (thumb *not* included) are bound together by muscle, tissue, and skin, they splint each other, providing added strength to each of the individual parts. When a fracture does occur, it is usually greenstick, hairline or impacted, but not displaced.

Finding a tender spot over a bone on the back of the hand is easy, but it may be difficult to know whether the tenderness is due to a bruised bone or a fracture.

One maneuver you may try is this: Have the patient hold his fingers and hand extended and stiff. Then sharply tap the ends of his fingers with a blunt object (i.e. knife handle, spoon, screwdriver head, etc.) If a metacarpal is broken, this sharp tapping will evoke pain *at* the fracture site, even though the blow is at the finger's end. You may compare the responses of different fingers, and the diagnosis will be apparent. Bone bruises of the metacarpals will not hurt when the finger end is tapped. (Fig. 4-11) A fracture will require professional help.

THE FINGERS

There are three bones in each finger and an intricate arrangement of tendons and ligaments that control their motion. Between the three bones are two joints which are the commonest site of injury to the fingers.

"Jammed Fingers"

Injuries that occur when a hurled object hits the tip of an outstretched finger, jamming the three bones together

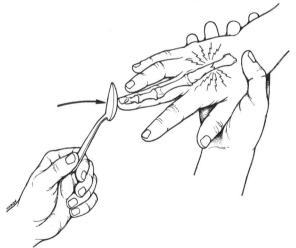

Figure 4-11.

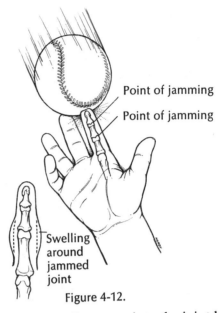

Point of jamming

Point of jamming

Swelling around jammed joint

Figure 4-12.

end-to-end. Bleeding usually occurs into the joint between the fingers, which produces pain, tenderness, limitation of motion and swelling. (Fig. 4-12)

Children usually call this injury after the appropriate sport from whence it came (i.e. basketball finger, baseball finger, etc.). However it is called, this is another good example of an injury that may be diagnosed and treated at home.

One first *inspects* the finger to be sure it is not out of place, deformed (other than swollen) and is straight. Then the patient is asked if he can move it. (This should be possible, albeit with some difficulty and pain.) Finally one gently *feels* the finger, bone-by-bone and joint-by-joint to ascertain the area of maximum tenderness. If the swelling and area of maximum tenderness are *between* bones, in the joint, a "jammed" finger is your most likely diagnosis.

It's quite important to make the diagnosis between broken finger and jammed finger, because the treatment is different. If the finger is broken, it should be splinted so that it is relatively immobile, for about 3 weeks. Your physician should do this, because the position of the splint should provide maximum comfort and utility.

But if it is a jammed finger, you should immobilize it with a splint for only a few days during the time of maximum tenderness. After that, the splint may be removed and the patient encouraged to use the finger, to loosen it up and hasten the absorption of the blood in the joint. On the other hand, the jammed finger may not require immobilization unless it is very painful when moved. In that case, immobilization will make it more comfortable for a few days.

If a fracture occurs at *the end* of one of the bones, (Fig. 4-13) a so-called chip fracture, maximum tenderness and swelling will occur at the joint rather than the midshaft and so resemble a jammed finger. When this is the case, the patient will resist early removal of the splint and

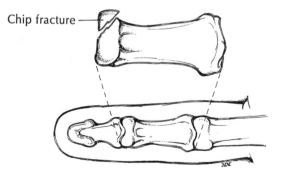

Figure 4-13.

continue to complain of tenderness which may be *on one side of the joint* rather than over the whole joint.

If this occurs, even though it may be a week after the injury, there's plenty of time to get an x ray, and, if it is really a chip, you will know to continue the splint for another couple of weeks. Not having had the x ray taken sooner hasn't done any harm, and the end result will be just fine.

Fingernails and Fingertips

The fingertip is especially prone to trauma. It gets caught, pinched, stuck, mashed, cut and banged in the most peculiar places and by the most incredible circumstances. There follows a list of injuries common to the fingertip.

Mashed fingertips occur mostly by being in the wrong place at the wrong time. Car and other doors, hammers and heavy stones or rocks are the offenders. The last bone of the finger is frequently broken, chipped or cracked in this injury, but this is of no consequence, since treatment is the same despite the presence or absence of a fracture. Pain and tenderness are universal and need to be dealt with quickly. Let us first discuss the finger that is *not* bleeding—that is, that does *not* have a cut or tear in the flesh or nail.

Ice the fingertip in a dish of cold water with ice cubes for 20 to 30 minutes. This will diminish pain and retard bleeding into the fingertip, which makes it tender and painful later on. If the child resists putting the finger in ice water, try to hold the *whole* hand in ice water for 10-15 minutes anyhow. (Fig. 4-14) Don't hold just the injured

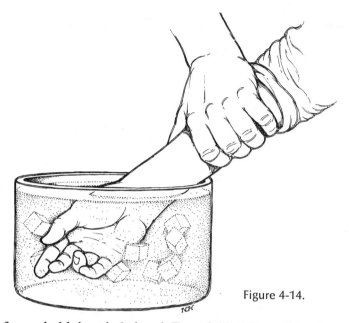

Figure 4-14.

finger; hold the whole hand. Forceful holding of the finger alone will retard blood flow and make for more swelling.

After the initial treatment you may wish to put a bulky dressing on the finger for a few days, just to protect it from being touched, which will be quite painful. (Fig. 4-15) But the most important thing to do is to apply a sling. The purpose behind the sling is to keep the finger, hand and forearm elevated. This will prevent throbbing and help reduce the swelling.

Don't feel that it's silly to put the whole arm in a sling just for the fingertip, and don't let your older child talk you out of it because he's embarrassed to go to school with a sling for a fingertip injury. Note that when he's *not* wearing the sling, he walks around with his elbow bent and his hand *up*. This is the position of maximum comfort, and you ought to help him maintain it!

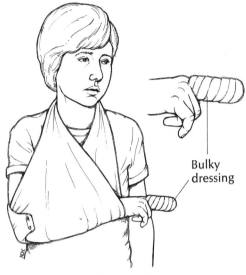

Bulky
dressing

Figure 4-15.

Bleeding Under the Nail. When the nail turns bluish-black immediately after a fingertip injury, there's been bleeding under the nail. This is important to ascertain because the blood may be under pressure and pain may be considerable! When this occurs, the blood should be drained. This will make the patient much more comfortable.

Although this drainage is not difficult, it had probably best be done by a professional. It should be done under relatively sterile conditions, because if there's a fracture of the bone underneath, drainage of the nailbed converts a simple fracture into a compound one (see above) and we don't want to invite the possibility of bone infection.

Further, there are several methods of draining the nailbed; your physician will select the least traumatic one depending upon the injury, the cooperation of the child, etc. He may elect to put a hole in the nail, or cut the cuticle, or even approach the collection of the blood from the side or the top. Let him do it. You'll be glad you did, and he will instruct you on aftercare.

Parenthetically, if blood is noted to be oozing from under the nail at one point or another, this bleeding should not be stopped but should be encouraged, as this will ease the tension under the nail. Gently and alternately squeeze the nail and the area surrounding the point of bleeding, in an attempt to "milk" the blood out from under the nail. When you've gotten as much out as you can, you will see some clearing of the black area through the nail. The tension will then be eased, and the area may be cleansed and a sterile dressing applied. And you've probably avoided a trip to the doctor *if* the patient is comfortable.

Most nails with *subungual hematomata* (bleeding under the nail) will eventually be lost and will be replaced by one just as good as the original. This, however, will take months. The new nail will push the old one out without difficulty, and in the process the exposed nailbed will *not* be tender.

Cuts of Fingers

Cuts of the finger and fingertip are treated the same way as other lacerations, with one *major* exception. Cuts of the shaft of the finger may involve tendons and therefore have to be examined *very carefully* for preservation of function.

When a child cuts a finger along its shaft, first wrap with bandages or a clean cloth and apply pressure to stop

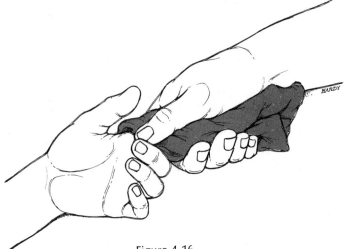

Figure 4-16.

the bleeding. (Fig. 4-16) After 15 to 20 minutes, when the bleeding has been stopped or slowed, the child *must* be encouraged alternately to bend and straighten the finger *(regardless of how painful this may be)* until you are satisfied that he can flex and extend the finger adequately. And I mean the *whole* finger. Even if it is only the tip that will not flex or extend properly—and even if the accompanying cut is less than one-half inch long—you must seek competent professional help if there is any question of loss of function! This must be fixed and fixed properly at the time of the injury. (Fig. 4-17).

Once you are sure that the finger's function is not impaired, you can treat lacerations of the fingers and tip like any other. If the edges of the wound can be brought and kept together easily, this should be done and a bandage applied. Sometimes the edges will stay together if the finger is kept straight, but when it is bent the cut opens

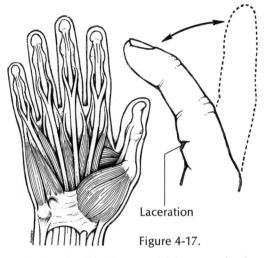

Laceration

Figure 4-17.

up. Then, obviously, the finger will have to be bandaged in such a way that it cannot bend. This may be done either with a bulky bandage or with a popsicle stick splint. (Fig. 4-18) The finger should be maintained splinted for two to three days and bandaged for a week.

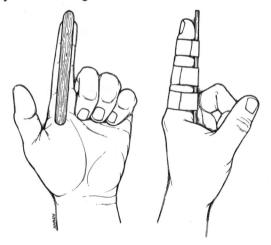

Figure 4-18.

Torn Nails

Torn nails hurt! This is one of the most painful fingertip injuries that occur, so you will invariably be dealing with a child who is quite upset, crying or hysterical. The first thing to do is to hold the finger firmly but gently, with a piece of cloth (to stop the bleeding and also to get the sight of the injury away from the child) and comfort the child! After this has been done, and the child is reassured (this may take a few minutes) tell the child that you are *just* going to *look* at the finger, and that you will not hurt it.

Now examine the nail carefully in good light and determine the extent of the tear. If it's small, in a straight line, and the nail or a piece of it has not been torn off, simply cleanse and bandage. The nail tear will not repair itself, but the wound will heal, and the tear will grow out without any trouble. You may have to keep a Band-Aid or piece of tape on it for weeks, however, so that it does not snag and catch onto clothing.

If, however, a piece of the nail has been partially torn off or pulled away from the nailbed, the torn piece should be removed. This is most easily accomplished *without* instruments. If the child sees you coming at him with a scissors or nail cutters, he'll take off! The simplest way to do it is to grab the torn piece of nail firmly between your two strongest and most dexterous fingers and *complete* the tear in the *shortest* direction. Barbaric as this may sound, it's the best way to do it, certainly the quickest, and will shorten the amount of time necessary to treat the finger before bandaging. (Fig. 4-19)

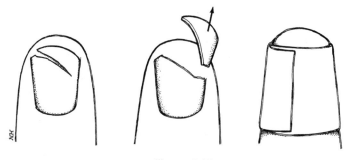

Figure 4-19.

If the whole nail has been torn off, one need only cleanse and apply a dressing. Sometimes it hangs only by a small thread of tissue. Remove the nail by the method described above. If the nail has obviously been mostly pulled off and then pressed back in place, you can't save it, so don't try. Take it off. As a matter of fact, I would remove *the whole nail* if 75 percent of it has been torn from the bed. One more second of pain now will save hours of grief later if you take definite action when appropriate.

Another good reason to take the nail off is the potential for infection. When nails are partially removed, the nailbed frequently becomes contaminated with dirt in the split second before the nail returns to its original position. The nail then seals the dirt in, and infection commonly occurs within a day or two.

When the nail is removed, cleanse and dress the area. A firm bandage will ease the pain, but the wound should first be dressed with an ointment. An antibiotic ointment would be preferable, but even petroleum jelly will do. This will keep the bandage from sticking to the nailbed. When the dressing is changed, if it sticks to the wound, it should be soaked in hydrogen peroxide. The bubbling action will free the dressing from the wound. Some of the newer Band-Aid materials are supposed to be non-sticking, but use the ointment anyhow. You'll be glad you did.

After a few days the nail bed will have toughened up enough so that only a Band-Aid is necessary. And when the nailbed is completely dry, the Band-Aid may be removed. The new nail will take months to grow, but it will probably be as good as the old one. However, it may not be, if the growth plate of the nail was injured in the original accident. This cannot be helped. Further it couldn't have been helped even if the injury were professionally treated from the beginning. So again, don't feel guilty. You've done as well as anyone could.

Slivers Under the Nail

A common enough problem, this condition is mentioned only to explore one ever-present hazard. Whether or not the sliver is removed, unless part of the nail is cut away too, the wound is quite prone to infection. It's as if dirt is *injected* under the nail and then sealed up and allowed to smolder.

Thus, a hole must be cut into the roof to allow the smoke out. A portion of the nail must be cut away so that the wound doesn't close at the junction of the nail and the skin. Invariably, the sliver will come away with the piece of nail. (Fig. 4-20) This may be done with a small, clean sharp scissors, will hurt for a second, and will then heal without infection. Soaking for 15 minutes, three times a

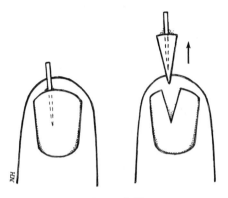

Figure 4-20.

day, will remove soreness, keep infection out and hasten healing.

FINGERS STUCK IN RINGS 'N' THINGS

Several times each year we are called upon to extricate little fingers from holes in things, or bigger fingers from rings too small. Sometimes the "things" and rings have to be cut, and there are devices available to do this without cutting fingers too. But there are also some tricks of the trade which you ought to know about, and which may save you a trip to the doctor's office.

First, never try to extricate a finger from a *sharp* object, or a finger which has already been cut in attempts at removal. The cut finger *proves* that the encircling edge is sharp, or has at least one sharp portion and the finger may be more severely cut by further attempts.

Next, it's important for you to know that the finger frequently swells *after* it has been encircled. This is why the object went on but will not come off. Also, invariably it's the first joint of the finger that stops the object from sliding off.

Here, in this order, are the things to try:

1. Lubricate the finger. Soap, cooking oil, petroleum jelly, any kind of ointment, kitchen grease, raw bacon—all these are good lubricants found in any household. Then try to remove gently.

2. If no go, insert the finger in a container of ice water. Slide the encircling object to a part of the finger where it's as loose as possible and begin massaging the finger from the tip upward toward the hand. You're trying to squeeze the swelling—the tissue juices—up past the encircling object. After several minutes, relubricate and gently try removal.

3. Last resort, and this works particularly well for too-tight rings, get some string or twine. The kind the butcher uses to wrap roasts is perfect. Slip one end of it through the ring, so that you have three to four inches *above* the ring, and several more inches *below* the ring. Now with the lower piece, begin to wrap the string tightly around the finger, starting right next to the ring and working down for about 1/2 to 3/4 of an inch. Hold in place tightly. Now grab the upper piece, pull down against the ring and you will note that an unwrapping process begins to take place from *above* the ring. You will need to unwrap the string *from above.* In so doing, keep pressure exerted on the string and ring in a downward direction. You will find that the ring begins to move down the finger, following the unwrapping string and sliding over the string still wrapped around the finger. (Fig. 4-21)

    You may have to rewrap and unwrap several

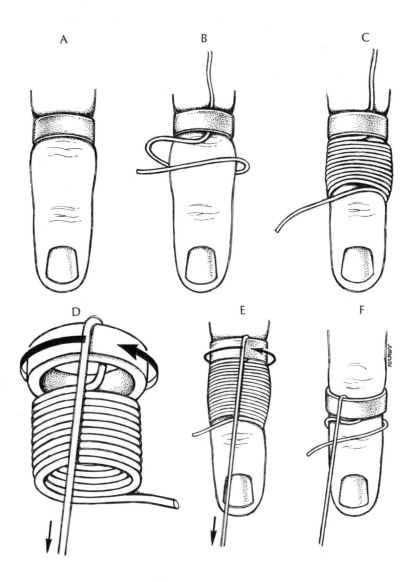

Figure 4-21.

times—and lubrication may help—but this method has saved many a ring from destruction.

Obviously, if this doesn't work—get help. And don't wait till tomorrow, the condition can only get worse.

5

Injuries to the Lower Limb

Running, jumping, kicking—it's a wonder that kids don't injure their legs more than they do. Nevertheless, leg injuries are less common than arm or hand injuries—certainly in toddlers. Later, when youngsters get involved more seriously in sports, the leg comes in for its fair share of trauma.

THE CHILD WITH A LIMP

This is a problem that occurs over and over again. The child, usually a toddler, for no explainable reason begins to limp. There is no history of trauma. At least, mother can't remember when the child fell, or otherwise hurt himself.

When one examines the child (and one should!) no reason for the limp can be found. There is no bruise, cut, abrasion or scraped area of skin; there is no swelling, tenderness, particular area of pain or discomfort, redness, black and blue spots or source of obvious infection. When the examiner moves the leg at all joints and in all directions no particular movement hurts. No splinters, cuts, burns—nothing!

The only explanation that I have is that the child has injured himself minimally and is undergoing deep muscle spasm. That hurts—it's what we call a "charley horse" or strained muscle. Further, since toddlers seem to tolerate minimal pain very well, they have a tendency to forget about their injuries. Consequently, they don't automatically protect their injuries as we do. They may even re-injure them over and over again, and this perpetuates the limp.

When I see a child with a limp—especially a toddler, and especially with this absence of physical findings—I have a tendency to "let them ride" for a week or two. I might suggest warm baths two or three times per day for 20 to 30 minutes, a heating pad (be sure the controls are on "low"), and sometimes a minimal dose of aspirin for a few days (the child's usual dose, limited to three times per day). I try to restrict their physical activity, as difficult as this is in toddlers, and I do a lot of watchful, hopeful waiting.

If the limp does not disappear in 10 to 14 days, a trip to the doctor is indicated. He may be more adept at examination than you and be able to focus on the specific area of discomfort. Or he may decide that some tests or x rays are in order. There are medical conditions other than trauma that can cause pain.

INJURIES TO THE HIP

Children rarely injure their hips. Other parts of the leg get hurt more readily, sparing the hip. However, it *is* possible to injure the hip, and when this happens, it is very quickly obvious that the patient requires professional care. Severe injuries of the hip usually involve fracture or dislocation in or very near the hip joints: the child is *obviously* severely injured. Pain makes the child inconsolable, the leg is in a distorted position; any movement elicits unbearable pain, and the leg may appear grossly shortened. (Fig. 5-1) Make the patient as comfortable as possible *without moving* him and GET HELP!

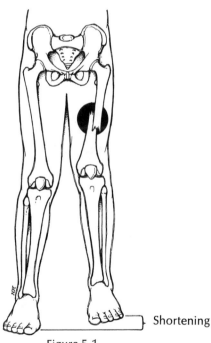

Shortening

Figure 5-1.

THE SPLIT INJURY

This is a gymnastics injury which is commonest in girls. A girl does a split and feels a sharp pain on the inside of the thigh, very high up—almost to the groin. Sometimes the pain goes away, and the child continues her exercises. However, an ache follows within 24 hours which doesn't go away.

She has certainly strained one of her adductor muscles, and is well advised to apply heat, hot tub whenever possible, take some aspirin and refrain from splits for a week or so. No permanent injury, no bad consequences, no trip to the doctor needed.

INJURIES TO THE UPPER LEG

There is only one bone to be concerned about—the femur. It's the biggest, strongest bone in the body. In older children who have had a chance to strengthen it with some years of weight bearing, it is very difficult to break and requires major trauma (automobile and bicycle accidents, skiing, etc.—accidents usually involving violent motion of the whole body). If weight bearing is possible, fracture is *not* a likely diagnosis.

The Fractured Femur

In infants and children under two years of age, the femur seems to break rather easily. An ordinary fall, a seemingly insignificant injury can do it. This may be caused by the lack of sufficient period of weight bearing to strengthen the bone.

The injury becomes apparent when the child refuses to move the limb and cries when it is moved by the parent. For some reason pain may be slight and the child may appear comfortable if left alone. The non-panicky parent will frequently watch the child for a day or so and may then note shortening of the leg. This is due to overriding bone ends, which become more so as time goes on because of spasm of thigh muscles. (Fig. 5-1)

The usual treatment is traction in a hospital setting, so of course, professional care is required. Unfortunately this treatment requires four to six weeks, so that the day or so you may have lost at the outset is not very critical. Remember, the important points are the child's total inability or even attempts to use the limb and then, possibly later, the leg becomes shorter than its opposite.

Therapy of Fractured Femur in Small Children

The following section might appropriately come under the heading of "pet peeve" and is of no practical value to the parent. But I take an author's privilege to describe one aspect of care which, in my opinion, needs change.

The usual mode of therapy for a broken femur in the infant under two or three years of age is to hang him up into what is called Gallow's traction for four to six weeks. (Fig. 5-2) This is a time-tested treatment to which the infant or small child becomes readily adjusted, cleanliness of the diaper area is facilitated and the results are uniformly excellent.

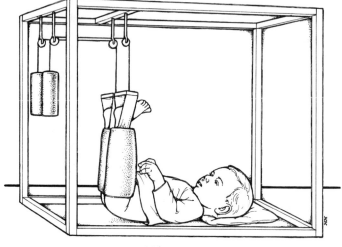

Figure 5-2.

So far, so good. My complaint is that *all* of this care is accomplished *IN HOSPITAL*. It takes a pediatrician rather than an orthopedist to understand the upheaval and chaos that the rest of the family suffers during this time. Parents (one or both) spend a major part of the day in the hospital, other children are neglected, either physically or emotionally, the breadwinner's job is frequently put in jeopardy, and the mother usually becomes exhausted.

I don't understand why, after an appropriate period, (several days to a week) during which time care of the infant in traction can be taught to the mother, x rays can be obtained to see that bone position is becoming acceptable, skin care is assured, the weights are adjusted and adequate circulation is documented—why the patient can't be sent *home!*

In this day of modern medical advances, why can't this infant, in an all-encompassing frame, be transported (you don't even need an ambulance, a van will do!)—set up at home and even brought back weekly for films and/or examination? Visiting nurses or home health aides could be sent in to check on the infant's condition—and, heaven help us, the orthopedist might even make a house call from time to time.

The savings and advantages of this technique, I believe, completely outweigh either the risks involved or the discomfort of changing time-honored practice and the convenience of the professionals involved. I have tried to sell this idea to numerous orthopedic surgeons without success. I really don't know why!

The Charley Horse

The commonest locations for a charley horse (strained muscle) are the upper arm and upper leg. There are so many muscles that either originate, pass through or end up associated with the upper leg or femoral area that it is not surprising that they occasionally get pulled, stretched, slightly torn or traumatized. This sets up pain, spasm, tenderness, and the charley horse.

Swelling is rarely evident—black and blue spots are more common. But almost universal to the diagnosis is the fact that the child, given proper encouragement, CAN BEAR WEIGHT. He can walk, although he may limp.

This is your tip that fracture, or more serious injury is *not* likely, and my frequent prescriptions of a tincture of time and some judicious neglect are appropriate. Of course, the time-honored routine of heat, rest and aspirin will facilitate comfort and hasten recovery.

THE KNEE

The knee is the site of an interesting paradox among childhood injuries. Although knees are among the most injury-prone joints in athletes, infants' and children's knees almost never suffer any internal traumas. In a recent excellent volume on childhood injuries for the medical profession * the knee joint is neither mentioned nor indexed!

So we don't have to worry about significant knee injuries in children below the pre-pubertal age range. Of course, they may occur, and when they do, they will be accompanied by readily noticeable swelling, pain and tenderness, and severe limitation of motion. Don't fool around! The injured knee *must* be seen by the physician. X rays are necessary to rule out fractures of the end of the long bones, and specific diagnoses must be made to ensure proper therapy.

Knee injuries in older children usually occur when the budding athlete gets seriously into such sports as football, basketball, soccer, skiing, and tennis. And the reason why the serious athlete *always* (almost always) injures his knee sooner or later is that he asks the knee to do more than the joint was ever intended to so.

Let's look at the anatomy. (Fig. 5-3) The knee is a "hinge" joint. It is only supposed to move in one plane or direction, and only through an arc of about 150 degrees (from 30 degrees to 180 degrees). But think about all the motions we make in fast stops and starts and sudden

* The Surgical Staff, Hospital for Sick Children, Toronto, *Care for the Injured Child* (Baltimore: Williams and Wilkins Co., 1975).

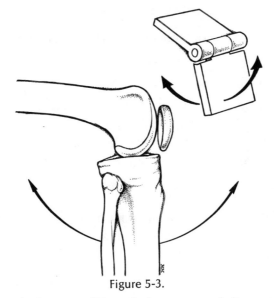

Figure 5-3.

directional changes. We ask it to extend its range of motion (stiff-legged activities to deep-knee bends), we ask it to rotate, and we even ask it to bend in directions (in and out, sideways) it's not built for. No wonder it gets injured so much.

I'm not going to encourage you to try self-diagnosis of knee joint injuries. It's too complicated, and the stakes are too high. With a *slightly* injured joint, *minimal* pain, tenderness, swelling and limitation of motion, a day or two of complete rest—with the leg elevated and a pillow under the knee so that it is partially flexed—is not unreasonable.

But if the injury is more severe, or if it doesn't get dramatically better in a day or two, it should have professional management for all of the reasons outlined above. Children have to live with those same knee joints for a lot of years, and knees seem to get more and more fragile as the years go by.

Painful Knees in Younger Children: One Warning!

In younger children (ages four to ten years) limping and knee pain may be related to a hip problem rather than the knee. The nerve distribution is such that pain may arise in the hip but be referred to the knee.

Here again, watchful waiting is in order for several days. But persistence of the symptom warrants not only a trip to the physician, but also films of both the knees *and the hips.* In this situation, if your physician doesn't include hip films in the evaluation, suggest it! Don't worry about hurting his feelings.

Painful Knees in the Adolescent (Especially the Budding Athlete)

It frequently happens that the pre-teen or teenager in the midst of a successful football/soccer/basketball/track season develops "painful knees." This pain is aggravated by training in sports and quiets down when the child is put to rest.

The physician's diagnosis may vary from "I find no evidence of disease" to highly technical medical terms such as *chondromalacia.* Varying degrees of rest, reduction or cessation of sports activity are prescribed.

And then we are in a "Catch 22" situation. The child wants to play. The parents are fearful of permanent crippling. Multiple opinions are sought and vary just enough in their recommendations that a hassle is set up between parent and child. Billy's friend Johnny has the same condition, and his doctor lets him play. The team gets into the state finals, and there's "just one more game."

What to do? A Solomon would be inadequate to the task! I have been involved in these battles many times and find that there are no set answers. Judgments are made based on the severity of the condition, the importance of psycho-emotional factors, the timing of the symptoms in relation to the length of the season, whether or not the team gets into the finals, etc., etc.

But I do ask both the parents and the child to face up to what I consider to be the really important facets of the decision. If we were talking about a "pro" whose livelihood depended on the decision, and in whom the decision might mean vast sums of money—that would be one thing. (Many of us might elect to play now and "fix" the knees later.) But we're talking about a schoolboy who probably *won't* go into professional athletics. This comparison often puts the judgment into more proper perspective.

PAIN BELOW THE KNEE—OSGOOD-SCHLATTER'S DISEASE

This condition used to be known as "housemaid's knee." It *was* more commonly seen in women who got down on their knees to scrub floors. However, with the lessening of that tedious task, and the increase in popularity of vigorous sports, it is now much more common in boys.

Young teenagers develop tender swelling of the tibial tubercle, the area just below the knee in front of the leg. The patient is frequently brought to the physician because some relatively *minor* trauma to the area elicits severe pain. Swelling is obvious. Although usually noted first on one side, it frequently affects both knees before long.

This problem is one of a family of many similar conditions that may occur in different areas of the body— the hip, foot, heel, spine, etc. And in each area the "disease" is known by a different man's name. The knee occurrence, however, is probably most frequent, and best known by lay personnel. (All the high school coaches and trainers are familiar with Osgood-Schlatter's Disease.)

Actually, it is an inflammation *(not infection)* of a growth center in the bone. It may be a thickening of soft tissue structures (tendons) and sometimes alterations in the apparent degree of calcification or mineralization of bone. (Fig. 5-4)

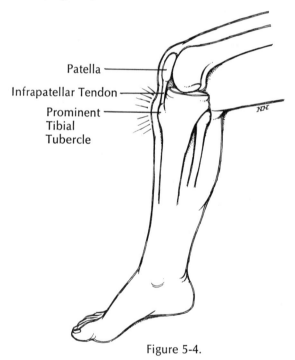

Figure 5-4.

Notwithstanding all these terrible-sounding names, the condition is benign and always gets better. It may last for months or a year or so, but is not usually very debilitating, and little if any treatment is necessary. I like to restrict deep-knee bends because I have an inherent fear of the child pulling the *infrapatellar tendon* off the *tibial tubercle* and having the knee cap end up halfway up the thigh—but I must admit I've never seen this happen.

Otherwise, I allow sports to the limit of painful tolerance and reassure the patient and parent that it always gets better. And it always does!

THE LEG BELOW THE KNEE

This portion of the lower limb contains two long bones, in addition to the usual muscles, tendons, ligaments, etc. One, the tibia, is large and bears virtually all of the weight. It also functions as the shin, directly beneath the skin, and makes up the inside ankle bone at its lower end.

The tibia is a tough bone to break. It requires a violent injury such as a skiing accident or skateboard injury. (I hate skateboards for this very reason.) Any injury to the tibia that makes weight-bearing impossible *requires* x rays and professional care!

Fractured Fibula

The other bone of the lower leg, the *fibula*, is a thin, weak-looking bone that traverses the length of the foreleg but bears virtually no weight. It is on the outside of the leg, and its main function seems to be to stabilize the ankle as the outside bone of the ankle joint.

It is mentioned here only because *rarely,* when the lower leg is *jarred* with considerable force, such as when the child jumps from a high place and lands on his feet, a loud, distinctive "crack" is heard, and pain may be felt all over the foreleg. Since the ankle is the greatest source of concern in this injury, films are taken of the ankle and lower foreleg, and they may be normal. (Fig. 5-5)

Nevertheless, force is sometimes transmitted *up* the fibula which can break higher up—above the view taken by the x rays. This child will continue to limp but may fool you because he *continues to bear weight,* albeit gingerly. Since the whole leg may be hurt initially, he may not be able to localize pain to the *upper outer* part of the foreleg. X ray of the area will reveal the fracture if there is one. They heal well.

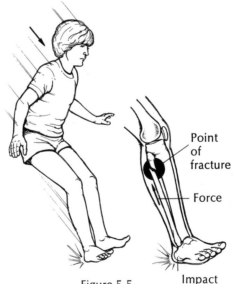

Point
of
fracture

Force

Impact

Figure 5-5.

Black-and-Blue Spots of the Shin

I see at least a half-dozen children per year, usually toddlers and small children, who present themselves with multiple black-and-blue spots of the skin over the shins. Parental concern usually centers around bleeding problems rather than trauma. Specifically, they're worried about leukemia.

Let me set this one straight right off. When children have a bleeding tendency—for whatever reason—they bleed all over! The black-and-blue marks are not limited to the shins but occur all over the body. So, black-and-blue marks on the front of children's legs are caused by bumps and falls, not bleeding per se, and are perfectly normal in this age group.

Two exceptions—both rare—must be mentioned. Persistent and tender bumps on the shins without black-and-blue marks should be brought to the attention of your physician. Also, hemorrhagic areas, black-and-blue marks on the legs but occurring front *and back, up and down* the legs, and not limited to the shins could be worrisome, especially if they look like bleeding *into* the skin rather than under it. This too is worth a trip to the office—but be reassured—if it is limited to the legs, the odds are overwhelming that we're not talking about anything serious!

Shin Splints

This may be a new term for parents, but shin splints

are well known to most junior high and high school athletes.

Shin splints are drawing, aching pains of the lower half of the shin, usually on the inside, occurring in athletes who do a lot of running. We see them mostly in kids playing soccer, running track and in running warm-ups for other sports. The actual cause of this discomfort is unknown, but it responds to heat, elevation and rest. Better conditioning usually causes them to disappear, and the athlete can resume his sport. No one ever died or became crippled from shin splints.

THE ANKLE

Another major trouble spot for trauma, the ankle joint comprises such a myriad of bones, joints, articular surfaces, tendons and ligaments that, like the knee, whole volumes have been written about this anatomical area alone.

Consequently there is no way that you can take care of any but the mildest injuries. So let's define a mild injury now: An ankle injury may be considered mild if there isn't much swelling, and if the patient can bear weight.

If either side of the ankle is markedly swollen, you're over your head, Mild swelling, the kind that you can notice only if you look carefully, can be dealt with. The mildly injured ankle will bear weight, although with some discomfort. The patient can be encouraged to walk, either on heel or on toe, or very flat-footed, without screaming pain. In the severely injured ankle, even the thought of weight-bearing will drive the patient up the wall. If you can't make up your mind about the degree of swelling, let weight-bearing be the deciding factor.

There are many reasons why I don't want you to treat ankles. Torn ligaments around the ankle are very common and may require a cast for complete immobilization. Complete cessation of weight-bearing may require crutches. X-ray films are necessary to find a chip or a small fracture that needs immobilization. The ligaments may be so strong that they have pulled a piece of bone off rather than tear. The patient should be carefully examined for injury to growth centers (epiphyses) which may not even appear on the initial x-ray film, but which should be suspected and treated at the time of the initial injury. For these reasons, and many more, you may treat the mildest ankle injuries, but for all the others—and when in doubt— get help.

Sprained Ankle

This is, by definition, the mildly injured ankle. To re-peat, swelling is minimal, and the patient *can bear weight.* Ice pack, elevation, relative immobilization (a pillow on a footstool) and something to relieve pain are all essential and should be done immediately. Continuation of this treatment for 24 to 36 hours will be helpful. (Fig. 5-6)

After the initial treatment, limited weight-bearing should be tried. The ankle may be strengthened by taping, by an elastic bandage, or by one of the commercial elastic ankle supports. A cane or crutches may be helpful. Elevation should be continued when the patient is not walking, and heat may be substituted for ice. (At this point you want to bring blood to the area, hasten resorption of

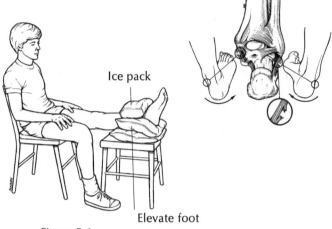

Ice pack

Elevate foot

Figure 5-6.

swelling, begin clearing away the blood under the skin and start the process of repair.)

If, however, the patient doesn't show dramatic improvement within just a few days, he should be seen by the physician for more careful examination and probably x rays.

Bike Fork Compression Injury

Picture an adult or larger child giving a smaller kid a ride on the cross bar of a bicycle. The passenger is not too careful how his or her legs swing, and one foot gets involved in the spokes of the rear half of the front wheel.

The foot is then quickly carried up to the bike fork and pulled partially through it. At this point the bike comes to a sudden front-wheel-braked halt and they both "wipe out." The passenger's foot may or may not still be in the fork of the wheel, but when extricated will frequently be

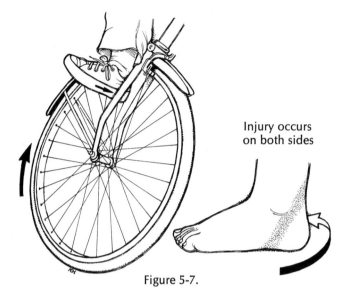

Injury occurs
on both sides

Figure 5-7.

found to have one or more crushing injuries in or about
the ankle. (Fig. 5-7)

The skin over the injuries has been crushed or
compressed. It is often white or bloodless, and the ankle is
quite painful. The child will not want to bear weight and
will be quite unhappy.

I urge you *not* to handle this injury. Crushed tissues
break down and die, slough out and need to be treated
very carefully, like burns. In addition, x rays may need to
be taken to see about the bones underneath.

So get help. You'll be glad you did.

"MARCH" FRACTURE OF THE FOOT

During World War II a syndrome which has come to
be called the "March" fracture was described. This story

was recorded on the medical histories of many recruits.

Soldiers would be taken out somewhere by truck. When they reached their destination, they jumped off the tailgate, usually with a full pack on their backs. On landing, they felt sudden sharp pain in the foot, usually most pronounced on the sole. A moderately loud accompanying "crack" might be heard. However, the pain was not severe, and so they started marching.

Shortly thereafter the pain would become very severe, and they had to stop. Back at the base, x rays would be taken which recorded nothing, and they were told to rest for a day or two. However, the pain continued. Without clinical or x-ray evidence of fracture they were not believed, were accused of malingering and some even ended up in the guard house. (Fig. 5-8)

Then someone thought of repeating the x rays after seven to ten days—and lo and behold, there was the

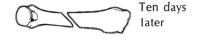

Ten days later

Immediately after injury

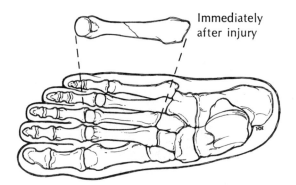

Figure 5-8.

fracture. These men had hairline fractures of one or more of the metatarsal bones; the fracture line was so fine that they couldn't be seen on the initial films. When the x rays were retaken later, dissolution of bone at the fracture line had begun as part of the normal reparative process and was readily discernible.

The reason why displacement of the bone ends does not usually occur is that the metatarsals are bound together by ligaments, and so splint each other very well. This also prevents much swelling, which could aid in the clinical diagnosis.

Moral of the story: If your child sustains an injury to his foot as the result of a jump from a relatively high place, and if pain persists for more than a few days—let him rest the foot for several days. Without swelling or gross deformity, you don't need to rush into x rays early. You may save the time, expense and radiation of an extra set of x rays by delaying the set for seven to ten days. But do have a set taken to ensure that proper healing is taking place.

THE PAINFUL HEEL SYNDROME

This is a form of the same injury that occurs to the tibial tubercle. In this location it is called Sever's disease or *calcaneo-apophysitis*. Occurring most frequently in boys between the ages of six years and puberty, it is benign and self-limited, but the patient has a tendency to complain a lot.

You may relieve his symptoms by putting soft pads, about ½-inch in thickness in both shoe heels. (Foam rubber, moleskin, molefoam, etc.) This should always be

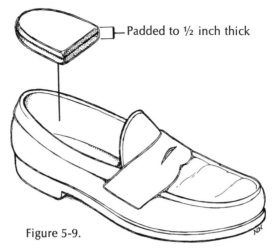

Padded to ½ inch thick

Figure 5-9.

done to *both* shoes, all shoes (even sneakers), and may have to be continued for a month or more. The treatment is inexpensive, may relieve his pain considerably, and should save you a trip to the physician. (Fig. 5-9)

TRAUMA TO TOES

Most often, toes are either stubbed, stepped on or have heavy objects dropped on them. If there is no bleeding under the nail (see this subject under "fingernails" above) and no gross deformity, it doesn't really matter *whether or not a fracture of one of the bones of the toes exists.*

The foot should be elevated to cut down on throbbing and ice applied to prevent swelling. Weight-bearing may be painful, but may be markedly improved by splinting the injured toe. (Fig. 5-10)

Toe splints are easy to apply and are very effective. The toe is simply taped to one or two of its neighbors. The first and fifth toes, if injured, are taped to the adjacent

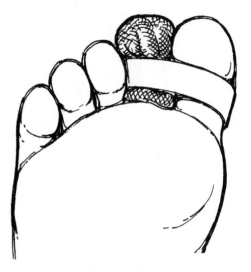

Figure 5-10.

toes. The second through fourth toes are taped to the toes on *both* sides of the injured one. However—and this is very important—a gauze, cloth or similar pad *must always* be placed between toes being taped together. This cuts down on perspiration, blistering and other skin trauma.

The simplest way to do this is to wrap the injured toe with a small piece of gauze or cloth. This eliminates the tape being directly in contact with skin; also, gauze pads or small pieces of cloth placed between toes frequently slip. Of course, it's wise and comfortable to wear toeless sandals or loose slippers while toe is healing.

The splint may be changed as often as desirable, and should be maintained as long as necessary for comfort. This simple device will provide comfort, save on the doctor's visit and obviate the x ray, which probably isn't necessary.

6

Head Injuries

This is a particularly important section for the do-it-yourself physician-parent; time, money, worry and x rays are expended most wastefully and most frequently in head injuries. I guess it's because there is such a large element of the unknown in head symptoms and such unwarranted fear of brain damage.

Let's set this one straight right now: I have seen perhaps a half-dozen instances of brain damage resulting from head injury in twenty years of practice, and I'm sure I've seen thousands of children with head injuries. In the few instances of serious head trauma the kids were so severely injured that there was no question that they needed emergency hospital treatment.

Most head injuries are quite mild. I have never seen a severe head injury in which there wasn't *gross obvious* physical evidence of the injury (unconsciousness, big bump on the head, marked area of black-and-blue discoloration—although this may come later).

RULE ONE—WHEN NOT TO CALL

Therefore, *Rule One*. Without unconsciousness, or a really big bump on the head, don't panic! You have time to observe the situation carefully and evaluate the child more thoroughly. A few minutes spent here may save you a lot of time, worry, expense and radiation later.

The head-injured child is immediately stunned, may have a few seconds of involuntary jerks or spasms, *doesn't* usually lose consciousness, is terrified, and cries lustily (although see "breath holding" below). After being quieted down, the child turns pale, may break out in a sweat, often vomits once spontaneously and may involuntarily wet or soil his underpants.

All of the above is *appropriate* behavior; these are symptoms and signs *reasonable* to expect of the head-injured child. *By themselves* they should not cause undue alarm.

RULE TWO—WHEN TO CALL!

On the other hand, *Rule Two*. If the child loses consciousness—however briefly—by definition he has sustained a *cerebral* concussion, and professional evaluation is mandatory. The only exception to this rule occurs if your child is a known "breath holder," or if the unconsciousness seems to be related more to breath holding than trauma. Let me explain.

BREATH HOLDING

Breath holding, as mentioned earlier, occurs in some infants and toddlers when they are suddenly startled or injured and take the first large breath associated with the beginning of a severe crying episode. What happens is that they take this breath and cry during the first long expulsion of air. Then the cry peters out. However, they continue to try to expel air, although there's no air left in their lungs. The attempt continues and continues and continues, but the child doesn't take the next breath. He turns blue, and then passes out. He may remain unconscious for a minute or more, but during this time *he resumes breathing* and his color returns to normal.

This is a fairly common occurrence among infants and toddlers and may be associated with any sudden traumatic or startling situation. Its importance in this discussion is to separate it from the immediate unconsciousness that means cerebral concussion.

HEAD INJURIES NEEDING MEDICAL CARE

Severe head injuries require professional care immediately. Parents should seek help in a controlled but urgent manner if the following signs or symptoms occur after a head injury:
1. loss of consciousness
2. convulsions
3. repeated vomiting which continues hours after the initial injury

4. bleeding from the nose or ears
5. severe, persistent headache, not relieved by aspirin
6. unusual repetitive movements of the eyes
7. unusual behavior, extreme sleepiness, inability to be roused from sleep
8. walking off-balance, acting "drunk" or falling to one side or the other, weakness of one side of the body

These are potentially dangerous symptoms which should alert you to get medical help immediately. Lacking the appearance of *any one* of these signs, and when the head injury appears mild, it may be treated in the following manner:

Treatment of Mild Head Injuries

1. Quiet and reassure the child. When quieted, look again for the danger signs.
2. If he will allow you, apply ice to the injured area in an attempt to reduce potential swelling.
3. Headache may be treated with an appropriate dose of aspirin. If necessary, this may be repeated every four hours.
4. Don't be in a rush to feed the child. Vomiting occurs easily in head-injured children; if you give him too much too soon, he might give it right back to you. Liquids are more important than solids, and small amounts administered frequently are more likely to stay down.
5. Allow the child to sleep if he wishes. He has to sleep sooner or later and I have heard stories of too many parents whose children injured themselves just before

bedtime and were then kept up most of the night because their parents were afraid to let them go to sleep.

6. Rather, awaken the child every hour or so for a few hours and then every four hours for the remainder of the night. You don't need to awaken him totally so that he's a problem to get back to sleep. Just be sure he's rousable, that he stirs appropriately, and that you could awaken him completely if you wished.

7. For a day or two after the injury he should be kept relatively quiet until all symptoms disappear and he seems his old self. When he fights hard enough over this forced inactivity, you'll know he's on the mend.

7

Trauma to the Face

Parents are terrified over face injuries; the possibility of disfigurement makes this concern logical. Yet the incidence of severe disfigurement is very low. Let's look at this concern critically, in the hope that the whole problem will seem less horrendous, and even frequently treatable at home.

In face injuries one is concerned about disfigurement as the result of lacerations and fractures of bone structure. Loss of function of the eyes, nose, and tongue is also worrisome. In some injuries, all of these factors must be considered, but most often they may be considered individually.

LACERATIONS OF THE FACE

Most significant lacerations of the face (those more than ½ inch in length, or that gape open) should be

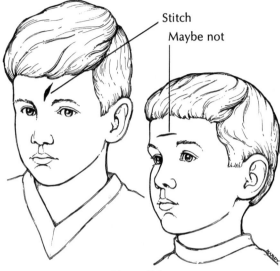

Stitch

Maybe not

Figure 7-1.

stitched. Scars of the face are very apparent and, in this age of beautiful people, undesirable.

Sometimes even smaller cuts will need to be sewn. Vertical lacerations of the forehead, because they are oriented at 90 degrees to Langer's lines, *always* scar noticeably and need all the help they can get. (Fig. 7-1) Conversely, horizontal lines of the forehead, especially if not too long and in a crease line, may fall together quite naturally and need nothing more than a Band-Aid or small butterfly.

Many people try to get away without sewing lacerations *under* the chin because they aren't noticeable. However, this may be a mistake. These lacerations are frequently "tear" injuries and therefore quite jagged and dirty. (Fig. 7-2) Also, an uneven, lumpy scar in this location will frequently be a source of irritation when this little boy starts to shave.

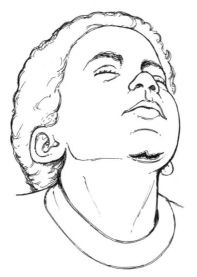

Figure 7-2.

Lacerations that fall naturally into crease lines may occur in areas of the face other than the forehead. Crinkle lines around the eyes are good places to hide lacerations, as are the upper and lower eyelids, the corners of the mouth and around the nostrils. These areas will frequently sustain small lacerations which do *not* gape, and which therefore do *not* need to be sewn.

Scalp lacerations under one inch in length do not need to be sewn for cosmetic reasons. However, stitches may be needed to control bleeding, since the scalp has a very rich blood supply. Also, if cuts gape significantly or are very jagged, they may scar badly and be a focus of irritation by a comb: this factor should be considered in the decision to sew.

Thus, the face and head offer some special problems which have to be taken into consideration, *in addition to* all of the factors outlined in Chapter 4. Be wise!

INJURIES IN AND AROUND THE EYE

Here is an area where we don't take any chances: eye-sight is much too precious. These are the direct indications for having a physician see your child without delay:

1. Any injury directly to the eye, in which you can readily see that the eye is injured.
2. Any injury *around* the eye or *to* the eye in which the white of the eye (the sclera) becomes reddened and stays that way for more than an hour or so.
3. Any injury that causes blurred vision in one eye, or double vision when both eyes are used.
4. Any injury that causes a painful eye.
5. Any eye that has a "foreign body" sensation that lasts overnight, especially if the sclera (white part) becomes and remains red all over.

To repeat, any of the above conditions *must* be seen by a physician sooner rather than later. Conversely, there are some eye conditions that do not have to be seen urgently and some that do not have to be seen at all. There follows a list of injuries that do not require immediate medical attention.

1. Ecchymosis (black-and-blue marks) around the eye, when *not* accompanied by any phenomena in the "must be seen" list can be just watched. Most kids with "a black eye" have no other injury.
2. Frequently as the result of hard coughing or vomiting a "red spot" of varying size may be seen in the sclera. (Fig. 7-3) There is no history of trauma, the rest of the sclera is not red, the eye is not irritated or painful, and

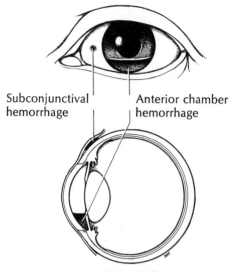

Subconjunctival   Anterior chamber
hemorrhage   hemorrhage

Figure 7-3.

vision is unaffected. This is actually a blood spot or
sub-conjunctival hematoma and it may be left to
disappear by itself. Remember, however, that this spot
must be in the white of the eye. Any blood seen in the
central portion of the eye, behind the cornea (the
window of the eye) must be treated as an emergency.
This child will probably have to be put in the hospital.

3. Small lacerations of the eyebrow, upper and lower
    lids, and the crinkle corners of the eye, which either
    fall in crease lines or which do not gape, can probably
    be left alone (after cleansing, of course) and will heal
    quite nicely.

4. Insect bites around the eye have a tendency to swell
    markedly, especially overnight. A child may go to bed
    with a small mosquito bite somewhere around the eye
    and awaken with the eye swollen shut. This is a
    natural occurrence and no cause for alarm. It relates

directly to the body's horizontal position in bed. The swelling will go down as the day progresses, but the following morning the eye may be swollen shut again. Antihistamines, generally given orally, may hasten the disappearance of swelling and may also alleviate any itching that occurs. (Constant rubbing will tend to prolong the duration of the swelling!) Otherwise, no treatment is needed, and the condition will cure itself in a few days.

All conditions not specifically mentioned above had best be seen by the physician. Or if an eye condition does not respond as described here, it probably should receive the benefit of professional care. As we mentioned at the beginning of this section, we take eye injuries seriously.

BLUNT (NON-LACERATING) INJURIES OF THE FACE

Features common to blows and other injuries of the face which don't break the skin are pain and tenderness, and black-and-blue discoloration. Swelling is always worse on the morning after the injury has been sustained, but by itself is not generally a cause for alarm.

When and when not to seek professional help, however, is difficult to define specifically and frequently depends upon the degree of injury, the symptoms and appearance. Some general guidelines are offered and then some specific warnings will be spelled out.

Severe pain that lasts longer than an hour or so following the injury frequently implies more than a minor bruise. Grotesque swelling may have the same implications. Interference of normal *function* of parts of the face should cause concern too; major rather than minor injury frequently causes this lack of function.

BROKEN NOSE

A broken nose is not common in children and is suspected far more often than it occurs. When present it will cause absolutely grotesque swelling of the nose, often closing and later blackening the eyes.

When the nose is broken it almost always bleeds from within. My therapy for nosebleeds is simple pressure, which does the job every time. Sit the child up and pinch both his nostrils closed with your thumb and forefinger. The pressure should be firm but not hard enough to hurt. Tell him to breathe through his mouth. The secret is to hold the nostrils pinched for twenty minutes *by the clock,*

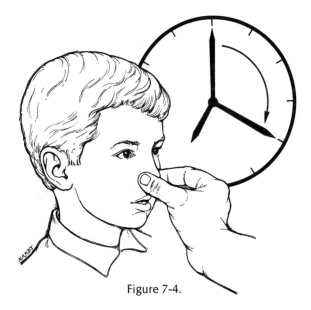

Figure 7-4.

without looking to see if the bleeding has stopped *during the entire twenty minutes.* (See Fig. 7-4) Every time you look to see if the bleeding has stopped, you disturb the clot, which may start the bleeding all over again. Clots frequently aren't firm for fifteen to twenty minutes.

This technique will stop most nosebleeds; the others will respond to a second twenty-minute period. Obviously this treatment may not work for older people with arteriosclerosis (hard _ing of the arteries) or hypertension, but for children it works fine.

Nasal fracture is rare in small children, because most of the nose is cartilage, rather than bone. (Fig. 7-5) Swelling on top or to the side of the nose rarely means fracture and can be treated with ice. However, if the grotesque swelling previously described is present, or if the swelling and ecchymosis get worse rather than better in the next day or two, the physician should be consulted.

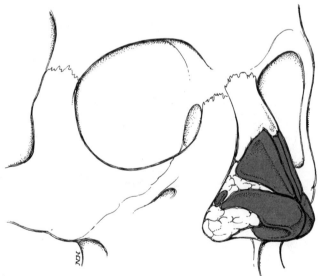

Figure 7-5.

FOREIGN BODIES IN THE NOSE

It is rather a common occurrence in small children to find foreign objects in the nose. For reasons totally unknown some children like to stuff things up their nostrils. Pieces of paper and tissue, small plastic parts of toys, beads, doll's eyes, berries, pussywillow buds—any of these objects are occasionally found in children's nostrils.

Sometimes they tell you about it, but more often it passes unnoticed for days or even weeks. Clues to the presence of a foreign body in the nose are recurrent bleeding from that side, a one-sided nasal discharge, and a foul smell from that nostril.

Take a look up into the nostril with a good strong light and try to see it. If you can see it you may be able to retrieve it if you're lucky, have a cooperative youngster and a smooth pair of tweezers. (Never put anything sharp into the nose!)

Try to grasp it with your tweezer—or if it's smooth, and your instrument slips off, try to get *behind* it and *pull* it out. A little bleeding may be expected, but if the blood flow is so massive that you can't see what you're doing, *quit and get help.*

If you are successful, remember that where there's one foreign body there's often another, so look again. And don't forget to check the other nostril.

FRACTURE OF THE CHEEK BONE (THE ZYGOMATIC ARCH)

This fracture occurs from time to time, and requires x

rays and sometimes manipulation. This diagnosis is suggested by severe pain, marked swelling and intense ecchymosis (black-and-blue marks). Sometimes if you press the area gently, bony ends can be felt to be grating against each other. Other symptoms that might be present are double vision and numbness of the gums on that side. See the doctor.

TRAUMA TO THE MOUTH

So many injuries may occur to so many of the structures of the mouth that they can't really be categorized. It's best to list them one by one.

Teeth

May be chipped, fractured, broken off, knocked out and discolored. Small chips require no treatment immediately. If permanent teeth, they may be capped for appearance's sake later. The same may be said for fractured teeth, if the fracture is a hairline one, and fragments are not loose.

Broken teeth may require care only because the nerve may be exposed, which is quite painful. When teeth, especially the two upper front teeth, are injured and bleed at the gum line, their nerves have often been severed. These teeth turn dark eventually and may need cosmetic capping if they are permanent teeth.

On the other hand, darkened *temporary* teeth require no treatment and should be left in place to act as space savers for the permanent teeth. When a child has a

Abscess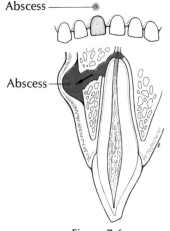

Abscess

Figure 7-6.

darkened upper incisor (front tooth) the parent should get into the habit of checking the gum above the tooth from time to time. These teeth frequently abscess, and you may see a draining pimple or gum boil in the gum above the tooth. (Fig. 7-6) Dentists often drain the back of these teeth, to cut down on infection in the soft tissues. Check with one.

When a tooth has been knocked out, if it is washed and replaced immediately, it often heals back in place. If the tooth is available, your dentist might want to try this technique and should be consulted. Unfortunately, this cannot wait until the next day; the dentist must be seen immediately.

Torn Lip Frenulum

The frenulum of the upper lip is the piece of stringy tissue that binds the center of the inside of the upper lip to the gum. It is sometimes quite thick and strong and may extend down far enough to separate the central incisors. (Fig. 7-7) Parents frequently ask me whether they should have this tissue clipped to allow the incisors to grow together. My response is to wait, because children frequently do the job themselves by falling on their faces and tearing the tissue completely.

This injury does not require treatment unless the bleeding won't stop. There's a good-size blood vessel in the frenulum which occasionally just won't stop bleeding. If this is the case, a stitch or two may be necessary. But before rushing off to the doctor, try ice. Ice pressed directly on the bleeding area or, if that's too messy, on the mustache area beneath the nose, may be helpful. Sometimes a child will let you press ice directly on the area, if you use an ice pop!

Lacerations of the Tongue

These occur frequently as a result of children biting themselves. They are usually small and most often will not require treatment.

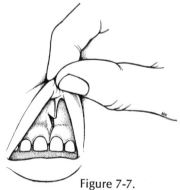

Figure 7-7.

Most lacerations of the tongue heal themselves with hardly a noticeable scar or deformity. Sometimes a small bump or irregularity remains, which is of no consequence. During the healing process, however, the cut will appear yellowish or contain pus. This is part of the normal healing process, and should not cause alarm. However, during this healing process the child will *not* appreciate food or drink that is spicy, contains citrus or which is salted or carbonated. It smarts!

Occasionally, when the bleeding of a tongue laceration will not quit (after *several* ice pops), or when the laceration is large or produces a large flap of tissue, professional help will be necessary. Fortunately, this is rare! (Fig. 7-8)

Other Lacerations Inside the Mouth

Healing occurs in the same way as tongue lacerations, in most instances. It is important, however, to examine them very carefully to see that they are not too deep.

After you've stopped the bleeding (several ice pops may be necessary), separate the edges of the wound gently

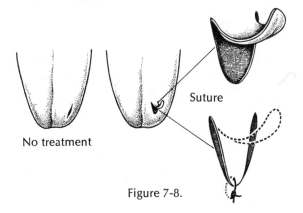

No treatment

Suture

Figure 7-8.

under a good strong light. Use your fingers or a cotton-tipped stick and try to see how deep the cut really is.

If you see anything stark white (bone) or very black (meaning very deep) you ought to let the doctor look at it. Or, if you can't adequately examine the area, let your physician do it. He may have to "insist" on the child's cooperation, which is sometimes difficult for the parent.

On the other hand, if you *can* determine that the laceration is superficial, it will heal in the same manner as tongue lacerations described above.

THE-ROUND-RED-MARK-AROUND-THE-MOUTH SYNDROME

From time to time a five- or six-year-old will develop a "rash"—a perfectly round, clearly marked, sharply edged circle of red skin, consisting of tiny skin hemorrhages, completely encircling the mouth.

No, he doesn't have a vitamin deficiency or some exotic disease. He was playing with a plastic cup or glass and held it up to his mouth, pressed it against his face and sucked all the air out of it. He then probably walked around with it clinging to his face for several minutes. The suction burst some tiny, superficial blood vessels on his face, creating the mark.

Leave it alone; it will go away. (Fig. 7-9)

THE JAW

The mandible, or jaw, rarely gets severely injured in childhood, although occasionally the older teenager will

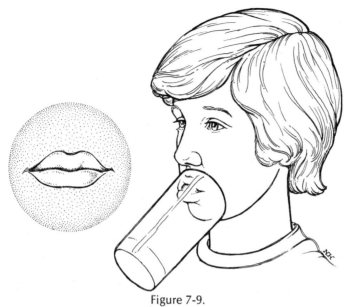

Figure 7-9.

have his jaw broken for him by some particularly skillful adversary.

Commonly, however, the smaller child will fall on, or get struck on, the jaw and have real difficulty opening his mouth. When the discomfort seems localized to the area *in front of the ear,* x rays frequently will have to be made.

The problem here is injury to the temporomandibular joint, the hinged joint that attaches the jaw to the skull. When this joint is "jammed," just as in fingers, swelling and bleeding may occur in the joint, resulting in severe discomfort and difficulty opening the mouth. (Fig. 7-10)

However, in contrast to the finger problem, this joint must be examined by x ray to be sure there are no fractures. Fractures in this area may require more vigorous treatment (immobilization) rather than just leaving them alone.

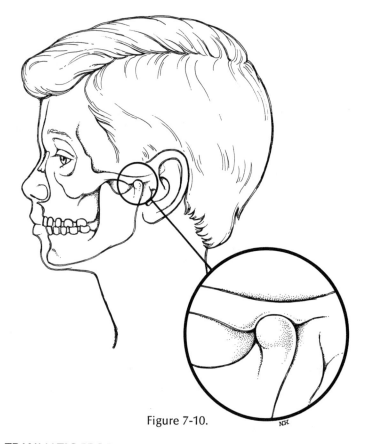

Figure 7-10.

TRAUMATIC PROBLEMS OF THE EAR

Once again, we're dealing with a vital sense organ, and in these four situations we *don't* treat at home:

1. Any child who has had a sharp blow to the ear, resulting in severe pain *inside* the ear or who is bleeding from the ear, should be seen by the physician.

2. Any child in whose ear you suspect that a foreign object (pencil, knitting needle, cotton-tipped applicator or stick) has been pushed, resulting in pain or bleeding, should be seen by the physician.
3. Any child who reports the presence of a foreign body in the ear, particularly if he has a history of inserting foreign bodies in peculiar places, or any child who has blood or pus discharging from the ear, should be seen by the physician. Don't try to remove such objects yourself.
4. Any child who has severe ear pain for *any* or *no* obvious reason should be seen by the physician.

Notwithstanding all of the above warnings, there are some ear problems that will get better by themselves. Bug bites in and about the ear may cause grotesque swelling but the ear will return to normal size and shape without treatment. Sometimes ice, or antihistamine administration by mouth, will alleviate itching and bring the swelling down a little faster.

Small, superficial lacerations of the ear will heal with amazingly little scarring, and may be left alone (after being cleansed, of course). Larger lacerations that distort the shape of the ear or that go through cartilage should be professionally treated.

INFECTED PIERCED EARS

As the fad for pierced ears has developed, so has an epidemic of infected pierced ears. Given the presumption that most of these girls follow instructions and keep their newly pierced ears clean, why do they become infected? I think I know.

I have seen a number of children whose infected ears have been swollen; with the skin actually grown *over* the clasp or small ball-type earring. This provided the clue. The children keep the clasp on *too tightly*. The clasp is pressed forward against the back of the ear and the front of the earring is pulled too tightly against the front of the ear lobe.

Thus a pressure *necrosis* (dead tissue caused by lack of blood supply from squeezing) occurs in the skin on both sides of the ear lobe, and it *becomes* and *stays* infected.

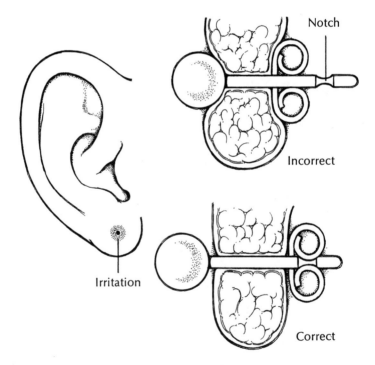

Figure 7-11.

The children do this because they don't want to lose their precious earrings—and they think that tight is safer.

Not so! Every earring post has a notch on it, way back near the end of the post. The clasp is supposed to set into that notch. That's where it's most secure. If the clasp is forward of the notch, it can actually *jump* the notch and be lost when the earring is pulled from the front.

So, mothers, warn your children about this. Keep the clasp in the notch where it's supposed to be. We'll have fewer infections and loser fewer clasps and earrings. (Fig. 7-11)

8

The Neck

Three types of neck trauma merit your attention. One is always serious, one may be serious, and the last, though quite painful, is never serious. Let's consider them in that order.

SEVERE BENDING INJURIES

These are injuries that occur to gymnasts, children playing on trampolines and divers who hit the bottom. The head is forcefully flexed, the chin strikes the chest and tremendous amounts of pressure may be exerted on the cervical (neck) spine. (Fig. 8-1)

The caveat or warning sign occurs when the child has difficulty moving an *extremity,* or feels numbness or tingling of any part of the body. Usually it will be in the shoulder or upper arm. The problem is potential nerve damage at its very root, coming out of the spinal cord,

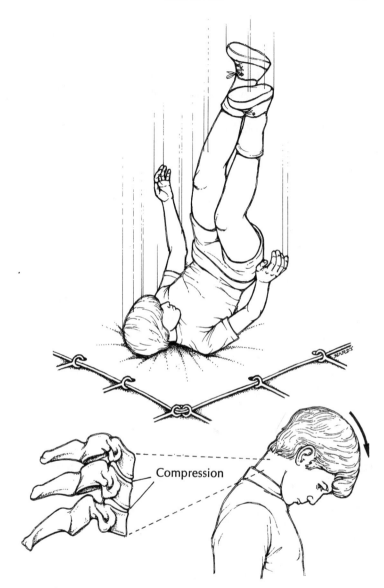

Compression

Figure 8-1.

because of compression of the neck vertebrae. This child needs to be professionally examined and x rays may need to be made.

As an aside, the severe extension of the neck that occurs in the so-called automobile "whip-lash" injury almost never occurs in children. They may experience the injury in the usual way and have a slightly stiff neck for a day or so, but there are never any of the residual effects that frequently occur in lawsuit-oriented adults. Hmmm!

BLOWS TO THE VOICE BOX

Children will occasionally sustain trauma to the front of the extended neck and complain of difficulty in speaking for a while. The loss of voice is not a problem, because the vocal cords are well protected. It must be kept in mind, however, that the larynx (voice box) is an integral part of the breathing apparatus and that swelling of any degree will cut down on the airway (such as occurs in croup). These children need to be watched carefully for signs of respiratory distress. (Fig. 8-2)

They will breathe more easily if their necks are extended, ice is applied to the external point of trauma, and if later they are put into a room to breathe warm moist air (from a vaporizer). Any sign of respiratory distress of more than the mildest degree, such as making noise when they breathe, should be brought to the attention of a physician. If they become extremely restless, if they seem to be working too hard when they breathe, if they get dusky in color, your physician should be called immediately.

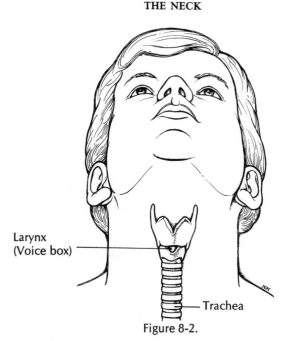

Larynx
(Voice box)

Trachea

Figure 8-2.

WRYNECK

An extremely common condition in children of all ages, wryneck or stiff neck (torticollis) occurs when one of the strap muscles (long thin muscle between head and body—there are several) goes into spasm or develops a charley horse. It is usually one of the lateral or side muscles, and therefore the head is usually pulled down to the side involved. (Fig. 8-3)

A child will frequently awaken with torticollis, without any remembered history of trauma, and someone will say he has a "cold" in his neck or has "slept wrong." When this happens, more often than not I have found that one of the lymph glands of the neck has been slightly swollen (as so often occurs in children for many reasons of little

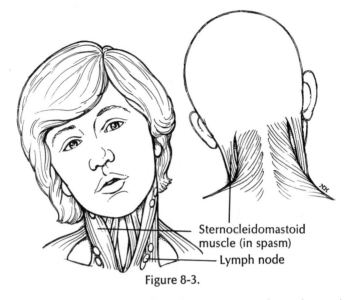

Sternocleidomastoid
muscle (in spasm)
Lymph node

Figure 8-3.

consequence) and has irritated a strap muscle and sent it into spasm.

These children always do well with conservative measures. When there has been an injury, ice early and heat later is the rule to be followed. Aspirin, as an anti-inflammatory agent, in adequate doses (don't piddle—if you're going to give aspirin, give it every four hours in the recommended dosage for size and age) will be helpful. You may use aspirin for a day or so, until the pain is better. If you need it longer, better check with your physician. The heating pad, and in older children, really warm, hard showers, with the water pounding down on the injured side of the neck, will provide immediate (though temporary) relief. They always get better in a few days.

In younger children, if you want to use warm baths, remember that you're going to have to have the water pretty high, and the child's head level pretty low, so DON'T LEAVE HIM ALONE FOR ONE INSTANT! These measures will allow you to cure most cases of wryneck without professional assistance.

9

Chest and Back Injuries

The chest and back house *vital* parts of the human body. Damage to the organs contained within can cause life-threatening and permanently crippling injuries. For this reason nature has evolved a bony cage around the chest and a bony tube (Fig. 9-1) called the spine, through which run the master nerves that supply the whole body. (Fig. 9-2)

It is therefore *very difficult* to injure the chest (heart and lungs) and the spine (spinal cord) seriously. Not that it can't be done, mind you. It certainly can. But it takes major trauma—a bad fall, an automobile wreck, a severe crushing injury—to inflict the kind of damage that can be life-threatening or paralyzing.

Most injuries sustained by children will *not* cause this kind of trauma. I have seen perhaps three or four children in twenty years who have had *significant* injuries of the chest, back or neck. Otherwise, in my experience, children get over these injuries very quickly and seem to be

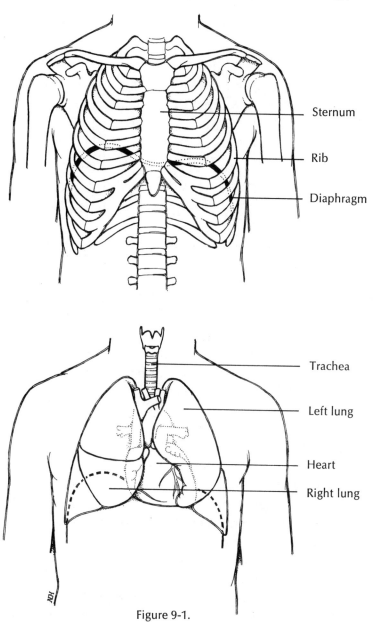

Sternum

Rib

Diaphragm

Trachea

Left lung

Heart

Right lung

Figure 9-1.

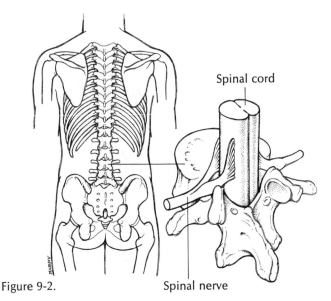

Spinal cord

Figure 9-2.   Spinal nerve

functioning without difficulty (albeit sometimes painfully) within a very few minutes.

Let us then get the dangerous situations out of the way—the warning signs of severe injury—and then learn how to treat the minor discomforts at home.

CHEST INJURIES

Before one can understand the dangers of chest injuries, one must understand something of the anatomy and mechanical working of the heart and lungs. The chest is a huge bellows. We expand the chest—literally make its capacity of volume larger—by lowering the diaphragm and opening up the spaces between the ribs. (Fig. 9-3)

When this occurs, the air pressure within the chest falls below atmospheric pressure, and air rushes into the lungs

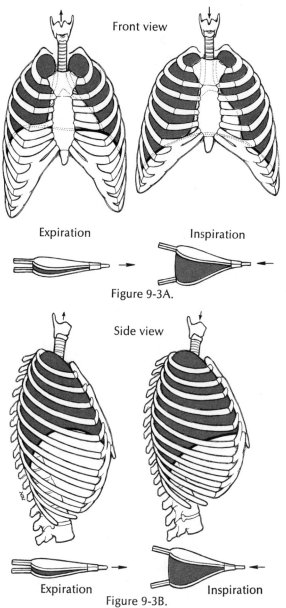

Front view

Expiration   Inspiration

Figure 9-3A.

Side view

Expiration   Inspiration

Figure 9-3B.

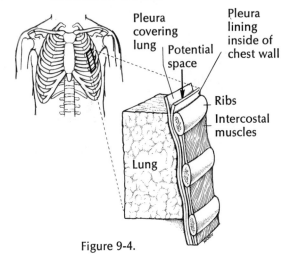

Pleura covering lung

Potential space

Pleura lining inside of chest wall

Ribs

Intercostal muscles

Lung

Figure 9-4.

(which expand as the chest expands). Then at the height of the breath, we reverse the process, elevating the diaphragm and narrowing the rib interspaces, which shrinks the chest volume. Air pressure in the lungs is now elevated above atmospheric, and air rushes out.

There is a *potential* space between the lungs and the chest wall called the pleural space. I say potential because in health the walls of the lungs fit smoothly against the walls of the chest, and no actual space exists. However, if anything gets into that space, such as air or blood or fluid—that pleural space becomes expanded by whatever substance is being introduced and can collapse the lung, since the outer chest wall is rigid. (Fig. 9-4)

Penetrating Injuries

These may occur as the result of a foreign object actually penetrating the chest wall (knife, sharp stick, iron fence railing, etc.). Or a crushing injury to the chest may break a rib which then penetrates through and into the chest. (Fig. 9-5) In the case of a foreign object penetrating the chest from the outside, during inspiration (breathing in), air may enter the pleural space from the outside. The chest wound may become a one-way valve, allowing air to enter with each inspiration but not allowing air to escape with expiration. Thus air will build up in the pleural space, compressing and collapsing the lung more and more with each breath.

This problem may be compounded even further by bleeding into the pleural space. It is also made worse if the lung is punctured, because that wound may be a one-way valve also, working in the opposite direction. (Fig. 9-6) Thus air may be entering the pleural space from within *and* from the chest wall, causing lung collapse even more quickly. In addition, the lung may bleed into itself or into the pleural space, making it even worse.

Wounds that penetrate the chest wall from the outside may be readily diagnosed. The sound of air rushing either *in* or *out* of the chest wound *makes the diagnosis!*

If this happens, plug the hole (your hand will do) until it can be bandaged tightly; call for help, and get the

Figure 9-5.

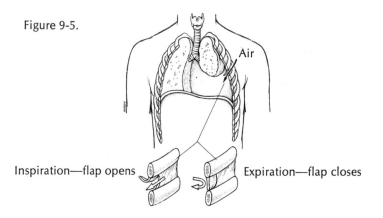

Inspiration—flap opens   Expiration—flap closes

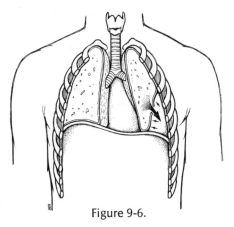

Figure 9-6.

patient to the *hospital,* not to the doctor's office. (Fig. 9-7) The emergency room is your best bet, and don't wait to call the doctor—just get to the hospital. In this situation you are justified in calling the police or an ambulance. You have a life-threatening emergency!

Crushing injuries may need to be treated with similar emergency measures. If a broken rib punctures a vessel which bleeds into the pleural space, or if the jagged rib end punctures the lung as described above, air and blood

Figure 9-7.

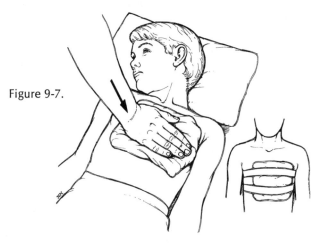

may be filling the pleural space and collapsing the lung. Here you will not have a hissing or sucking wound of the chest, but you may see increasing difficulty in breathing; unrelenting cough (this makes the breathing even more difficult); short, shallow, rapid respirations or skin color turning ashen, dusky or even blue. Don't wait—get help fast!

These life-threatening situations—penetrating and/or crushing injuries of the chest—are *quite rare* and only occur with *very* severe trauma. What *does* happen more often is that with a moderately severe, blunt blow to the chest, the child will get "the wind knocked out of him." He will get frightened, may attempt to cry and will appear *instantly* to have trouble breathing.

Without severe injury, *without* an obvious sucking or hissing chest wound, *without* duskiness or a blue discoloration to the skin, *without* increasing difficulty breathing, one can usually spend a few minutes of watchful waiting and see the patient improve in a very short time. This is what usually happens, and your anxious minutes spent in waiting will pay off.

Broken Ribs (Non-Penetrating)

This also is very rare in childhood, because the youthful rib cage is quite flexible. The patient who has a bruised, injured or even broken rib will not have difficulty in breathing, but will *not* want to take very deep breaths because it hurts. He will therefore have short and shallow respirations, he may grunt with each one, but he won't be breathing rapidly, he won't be having any trouble moving air and his color will be good.

He too may profit from a period of watchful waiting. In this situation, if improvement continues over minutes and then hours, he might not even need x rays to diagnose rib fracture. Without a specific point of tenderness on the rib cage—and especially in a prepubescent child with a highly pliable rib cage—fracture is highly unlikely. He will probably get better all by himself.

BACK INJURIES

Believe it or not, serious back injuries almost *never* occur in children. Certainly I've never seen one in a prepubertal child. By serious, of course, I mean injuries to the spine with a potential for nerve damage or paralysis. Most childhood back injuries are simple sprains or strains which get better with time, the heating pad, warm baths and aspirin.

And such injuries never seem to lead to chronic back syndromes, the kind that plague old crocks like us. The little guys and gals get injured, are stiff for a few days and then get better. Simple as that.

To Move or Not to Move

Most children with back injuries may be moved to make them more comfortable or to get them out of the traffic, wet, snow, or vomitus. The best way to approach this problem is to see if he can move his extremities. These rules have been fully discussed in Chapter 1, but a brief summary of that information is repeated here for convenience. (Fig. 9-8)

Move if:

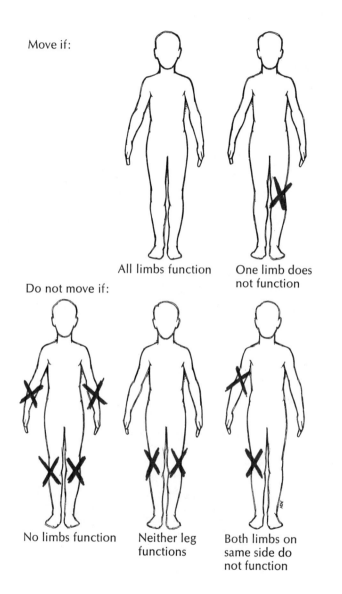

All limbs function   One limb does
not function

Do not move if:

No limbs function   Neither leg   Both limbs on
functions   same side do
not function

Figure 9-8.

1. All four limbs function—OK to move.
2. One limb doesn't function, immobilize that limb and move.
3. DO NOT MOVE IF:
    a. no limb functions
    b. neither leg functions
    c. both limbs on the *same* side do not function

These are rare circumstances, so rare as to be almost theoretical. Most children can be moved so as to be made more comfortable!

KIDNEY TRAUMA

This occurs in a small percentage of children that injure their backs low down, just above the buttocks, and on one side or the other, never directly in the middle of

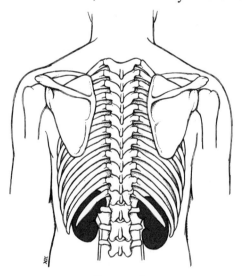

Figure 9-9.

the back. (Fig. 9-9) Even this injury usually gets better without specific treatment most of the time. However, the diagnosis *must* be made, and then the patient *must* be followed carefully.

To play it safe, if a child has a low, one-sided back injury with pain and tenderness that persists longer than an hour or so, collect the next specimen of his or her urine and look at it. Traumatized kidneys usually bleed, and the blood will tinge the usual yellow color pink or even red. If this occurs your doctor should be notified, and he'll probably want to look at the urine and the child.

If he detects blood in the urine, either grossly (visible to the naked eye) or by chemical or microscopic analysis, he'll probably want to continue to look at daily urine specimens to check progress. Most of these traumatized kidneys heal themselves over the course of several days, but your doctor will have to keep tabs on the urine and the patient.

10

Blows to the Belly

There are some particularly troublesome areas in the belly which are prone to serious trauma. Mostly, however, blows to the belly are more "bark than bite." The so-called "solar plexus" is really the *celiac plexus,* a coming-together of nerve junctions which are then distributed to the various organs of the abdomen. Thus, a blow to the solar (celiac) plexus can have ramifications in many different abdominal organs.

When a blow occurs, particularly in the very center of the stomach, a series of "visceral" (relating to stomach structures or organs) reactions occur. There is immediate pain, usually a reflex doubling over, and then a rapid shock-like state. The patient (or should I say "victim") becomes pale, gets sweaty, may turn green or gets sick to his stomach, may vomit or soil his underpants and gets very weak.

Fortunately this is all that usually happens. Since there are no very rigid organs in the center of the stomach, they move with the blow and usually are not damaged. The patient, after a few moments of discomfort, gets better, and that's usually all there is to it.

THE TRIANGLE OF TROUBLE

However, outside the center of the abdomen one encounters what I call the *triangle of trouble*—the liver, spleen and bladder. (Fig. 10-1) All of these organs may be seriously traumatized, even ruptured or torn. Although, it usually takes some pretty severe trauma from a bicycle or sled mishap, on a football field or as the result of a motor vehicle accident. In my experience this sort of trauma

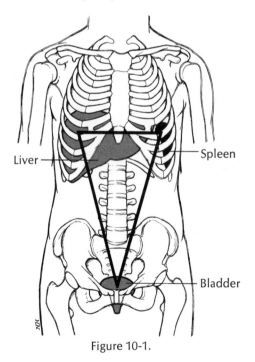

Liver — Spleen

Bladder

Figure 10-1.

occurs most frequently in older children and young teenagers, probably because only older children generate the kind of momentum in their activities that is necessary for blows of this severity.

As you can see by the diagram, blows to any area of the upper abdomen can mean trauma to the liver or spleen. On the left, the spleen is usually involved and on the right, the liver *may* be affected, although this seems to be a hardier organ than the spleen.

Trauma to the Spleen

Usually results in a rupture or tear; when that occurs there is bleeding into the abdominal cavity or peritoneum. This causes pain (often radiating to or felt in the left shoulder) and shock (pallor, sweating, nausea, weakness) *that persists* and which requires *urgent professional care.*

Don't hesitate on this one. Being fooled by a false alarm is much preferable to "waiting a little longer." Any trauma to the left upper quadrant that causes severe persistent pain or any symptoms described above represent a bona fide emergency until proven otherwise!

The treatment of ruptured spleen is surgical removal (although recently there have been attempts at repair). We'll leave this one to the surgeons. They're best equipped to make these judgments.

Trauma to the Liver

Could read just like the section on trauma to the spleen. However, the liver is less likely to be ruptured or torn or to bleed, so the odds are with you. When severe injury does occur, and if the symptoms described above are present, get the child to a hospital as soon as possible. Severe trauma to the right *upper quadrant* may have the same implications for the liver as the left upper quadrant for the spleen. Don't wait—get help fast.

Trauma to the Bladder

Children frequently "hold"their urine for long periods of time—they're just too busy to relieve themselves. This may distend the bladder to the point where it loses the protection of the pubic bone. (Fig. 10-2)

A fall or blow to the lower abdomen, when the bladder is distended, could conceivably rupture it. I put this injury into the theoretical category because I have never seen it occur as an isolated injury. However, it has been reported, and so I feel that it should be mentioned.

Symptoms would include severe pain in the center of

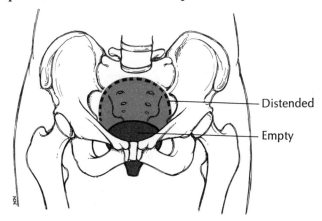

Distended

Empty

Figure 10-2.

the lower abdomen and bloody urine, although the child might not urinate for several hours. This condition requires surgical intervention.

In summary then, the overwhelming majority of blows to the belly will not be consequential. Symptoms will be only transient, and the patient will improve rapidly.

However, when symptoms persist, when their location is in the "triangle of trouble," or when they resemble symptoms described above, help should be sought urgently. If in doubt, it's better to be safe than sorry!

11

Injury to the Genitalia

Serious injury to the genitalia of either gender, fortunately, is quite rare. Boys, with organs more exposed and accessible, are at greater risk. Although girls are almost never seriously injured, they cause more concern because of concepts of anatomical virginity.

FEMALE GENITAL INJURY

The little girl child falls straddling something. a wall, a fence, a log, a toy. Her underpants become blood-tinged and she complains of pain "in her bottom." Believe it or not, this is as far as parents or surrogate parents (teachers, baby sitters, friends, etc.) ever get.

Sometimes a parent will remove the underpants and put the child in a lukewarm tub. But they don't examine the child. Why? Sometimes they don't want to, for fear of what they may find. Sometimes the child won't let them—

either because of the same fear, or because it hurts.

I have examined dozens of these frightened, hurt children, and invariably I find the same thing: a bruise, and a very small cut or tear in the labia. (Fig. 11-1) It is never serious, never requires anything more than the most conservative care, and always gets better with lukewarm tub baths three to four times per day for 15 to 20 minutes at a time.

Of course, one should never say "never" in medicine. The occasional severe injury does occur. But the odds on it *not* occurring are so good that you owe yourself at least the benefit of a good look at the wound before panicking. The criteria for sewing up significant lacerations are the same as described in Chapter 4. (But cosmetic appearance is almost never a problem.)

One possible problem, even in the simple labial laceration: Urination may be unpleasant, since urine may burn the bruised or cut area. If this occurs, and the child

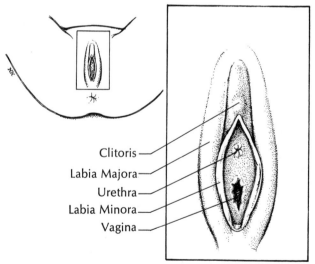

Clitoris
Labia Majora
Urethra
Labia Minora
Vagina

Figure 11-1.

then tries to retain urine, put her in a tub of lukewarm
water and encourage her to urinate right in the tub. Her
urine will be instantly diluted and she will experience no
discomfort. She may then be bathed in fresh water.

MALE GENITAL INJURIES

Little boys get their penises caught *under* the toilet seat
and in zippers. Never seriously. Zippers cause small cuts
or lacerations which require only good hygiene. Toilet
seats cause bruises which get better. Occasionally, swelling
makes urination difficult, but the warm tub trick works
here too.

Torsion of a Testicle

One problem does occur in older boys which may
require urgent action.

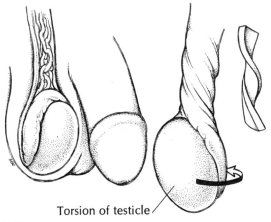

Torsion of testicle

Figure 11-2.

Occasionally as the result of trauma, but more often for no discernible reason, an older child (just pubertal or late prepubertal) will develop severe pain in one testicle (testis). On examination the testis is tender, may be swollen and slightly discolored.

It is possible that the stalk or cord of the testicle has become twisted, thus endangering the blood supply to it. (Fig. 11-2) This constitutes a genuine emergency, since a few hours of delay could damage the testicle beyond recall.

This is a matter for your physician, who should be called immediately. Don't worry about "crying wolf" on this one.

12

Thermal Injuries—Burns and Frostbite

Thermal wounds occur when skin is injured by extremes in temperature—too hot or too cold.

TYPES OF BURN INJURY

Burns may occur to skin in a variety of ways. *Flame* burns are obvious. *Radiation* burns occur from radiated heat, such as extreme sunlight, actual atomic radiation, or closeness to a very hot object. If the hot object is touched, this is a *contact* burn. When the hot contacting object is liquid, we have a *scald* burn.

Other more esoteric burns occur. *Chemical* burns injure the skin by heat or other destructive action. One must be quick to wash the chemical off; as long as it is present, the skin continues to be injured. *Friction* burns are notorious for dirt and foreign material ground into the skin. These wounds must be carefully cleansed, lest the foreign bodies (particles of dirt or minute slivers of wood or rope fiber) remain in the skin and cause a tattoo effect after healing. *Electrical* burns are sneaky because the damaged area frequently extends to a depth never anticipated. Actually, the burned area may be anywhere between the two points of contact of the electricity.

The two points of contact are *not* the two prongs of a plug, or the two holes of a duplex outlet. They are (1) the electrical source (either of the above) and (2) the part of the body that is grounded.

SEVERITY OF BURNS

First-Degree Burns

A diagram of normal skin is illustrated in Fig. 12-1a. First-degree burns cause redness of the skin. Most sunburn is a first-degree burn. Pain may be severe, but blisters do *not* occur. These burns are superficial, involving only the outermost layer of skin. They may peel later, but are essentially harmless. (Fig. 12-1b)

Two exceptions. First-degree burn over most of the body can be quite debilitating. In addition to the obvious discomfort of the injured skin, this patient may exhibit signs and symptoms of heat intoxication. Fever, headache, vomiting and generalized miseries may all be present. Aspirin, rest, liquids, added salt to the diet and local skin lubrication will all be helpful.

Second, any burn of the eyes warrants professional attention. The best example is the teenager trying to cure acne, who falls asleep under the sunlamp. A physician must be consulted about any child (or adult) who has painful, red, teary eyes following severe sunburn of the

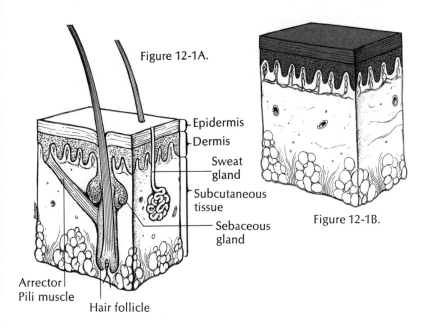

Figure 12-1A.

Epidermis
Dermis
Sweat gland
Subcutaneous tissue
Sebaceous gland

Figure 12-1B.

Arrector Pili muscle

Hair follicle

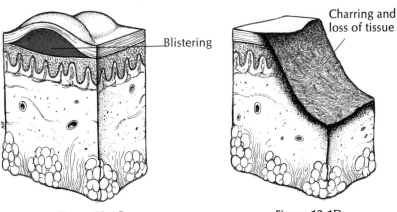

Blistering

Figure 12-1C.

Charring and loss of tissue

Figure 12-1D.

face. A careful evaluation of the degree of injury and appropriate treatment must be started.

No child (of any age) should be allowed to use a sunlamp unless *another* person is in the house and has been charged with the responsibility of checking on the sun worshipper frequently. Teenagers fall asleep so easily!

Second-Degree Burns

There is immediate or almost immediate blistering. The outermost layer of skin has been destroyed, and a significant portion of the body of the skin has been injured. (Fig. 12-1c)

It is possible, by estimating what percentage of the skin surface has sustained second-degree burns, to prognosticate how sick the child will be. And you can estimate what percentage of skin surface is burned by using the following scheme;

THE RULE OF NINES. If one assigns values of nine (9), or multiples thereof, to the varying parts of the skin surface, one may come up with a useful estimate of percentage of skin surface burned. (Fig. 12-2)

Head	9% x 1 =	9%
Each arm	9% x 2 =	18%
Each leg	18% x 2 =	36%
Torso	36% x 1 =	36%
Genitals	1% x 1 =	1%
		100%

One must remember that arm values may be divided

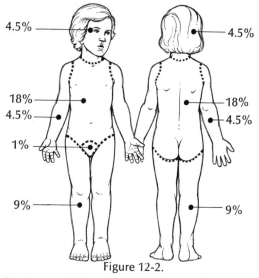

Figure 12-2.

in half for front and back sides, as may the legs. And the torso may be divided four ways (upper and lower, front and back) for purposes of easier and more exact calculations. Actually, this method is more accurate for adults (individuals 15 years of age or more) but for our purposes, this "guesstimate" is close enough.

After you've estimated the percentage of skin surface with second-degree burns, here are the guidelines for your responses:

1. Children with burns of more than 5 percent of their skin surface should be seen by your physician! He may allow you to care for this child yourself, but he will surely need to prescribe the treatment!

2. Children with burns of more than 10 percent of their surface area will probably need hospital care for intravenous fluid therapy, professional skin care, antibiotics and special dressings.

3. For children with 30 percent or more of their skin surfaces sustaining second-degree burns, transportation to a *burn center* (a hospital specializing in burn victims) represents optimum therapy. These children will be sick, sick, sick! *(Although this may not be obvious at the time of the initial injury.)*
4. Children with burns over more than 50 percent of their bodies will have great difficulty surviving, even with the best care.

It isn't often in this book that I've used "scare tactics," but I make no apologies for it here. Burns can be horrendous, life-threatening injuries in children. Your professionals are well trained! Use them!

Third-Degree Burns

Are full-thickness burns of the skin. The most severely affected areas of a third-degree burn will be white in color (no life) or black (charred). There will be no pain in this area, because there are no viable nerves left to carry pain sensation. (Fig. 12-1d)

All third degree burns will scar!

All third degree burns, if extensive enough, will need skin grafts!

All third degree burns will require professional care!

HOME TREATMENT OF BURNS

Notwithstanding all those warnings, significant burns requiring hospital care, or even professional care, are few.

Most burns are small, well under 5 percent of body surface, and not third-degree. Therefore they may be safely handled at home.

The rapid immersion of a superficial burn in cold water not only makes the burn feel better but immediately stops the further destruction of tissue. This should be done fast, for 15 to 20 minutes, after which a better evaluation and a decision on treatment can be made.

Two general methods have been described in the management of burns; their difference relates to whether or not permanent dressings are applied. As you will see, different circumstances make one or the other more appropriate.

Closed Treatment

Basically the burn is copiously and meticulously cleansed. PHisoHex soap is particularly appropriate because it is liquid and antibacterial. The burned area is gently dried with a very clean cloth or gauze pad (sterility is preferable). Large amounts of an antibacterial ointment (Bacitracin Neosporin) are applied. This ointment further prevents infection and will keep the oozing flesh from sticking to the dressing. Then the dressing. Many layers of sterile gauze pads followed by many wraps of rolled gauze.

The final dressing should be firm—not tight—bulky, and it generally will make the wound feel better. This type of dressing will be applicable mostly to hands and feet, portions of arms and legs and smaller burns of the torso. The dressing should be quite comfortable and may usually be left in place for 3 to 5 days. If it begins to unwrap, become dirty or slips so that the wound is exposed, it should be added to rather than rewrapped unless it's time for another dressing.

When the dressing is removed for changing, some areas may stick to the wound. This may be soaked loose, preferably with hydrogen peroxide, but lukewarm water will do. The same treatment is then provided; meticulous and copious washing with pHisoHex soap and lukewarm water, gentle removal of dead skin, patting dry, antibiotic ointment and the dressing.

These dressings may be changed about twice weekly. Since the wound usually heals from its outer edges inward, the dressing will get progressively smaller. Do not fall into the trap of using adhesive tape, as this injures tender new skin. When the skin has completely healed, it will have a smooth shiny surface of new dry skin and be non-tender, although still red. At this point, dressings may be discontinued. You've done a good job!

Open Treatment

The open treatment of burns is reserved for areas that are continually contaminated, such as the diaper area—areas where the likelihood of infection is very high. You won't want to close such a wound up for several days at a time. Open treatment is also used in places difficult to bandage (such as the face) and in extensive burns where bandaging would be difficult and painful. Some skin surface needs to be kept open for examination and treatment, although these are mostly hospital cases.

In these situations, either no bandage is used, or easily launderable articles of clothing may be worn such as Tshirts, underpants or socks. Again, dead skin, old blisters, etc. are removed meticulously and the area is cleaned with pHisoHex soap and water, gently patted dry and liberally spread with an antibiotic ointment.

The wound is then either left open, or a loose article of apparel is applied to act as a dressing. Obviously this wound must be cleansed more frequently, every day or so, and—the article of clothing may have to be soaked before it comes off. The basic treatment works well, and the burn heals in approximately the same amount of time.

MOTORCYCLE BURNS

There is nothing special about a motorcycle burn except its size, shape and location. Usually second degree, it may be imbedded with some foreign material (clothing—pant leg, etc.) and responds to the usual treatment of

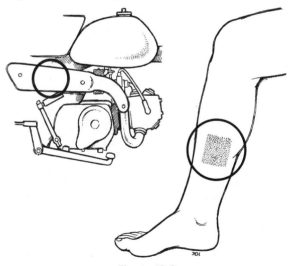

Figure 12-3.

cleanliness, antibiotic ointment and a dressing. (Fig. 12-3) However:

1. It's always on the inside of the calf.
2. It's always square.
3. It's always about 2x2 inches in size.

The burn comes from riding, usually as a passenger, on a motorcycle, and having one's calf touch an unprotected muffler. If you allow your kids to ride on motorcycles, this is one of the hazards. If you've forbidden it—this should be all the evidence you need.

FROSTBITE

The other type of thermal injury, frostbite, is much less common and also less apt to cause severe injury than burns. Notwithstanding all the stories we've heard of people losing fingers and toes from frostbite, it rarely occurs.

More often, we see children with cold injuries less severe than frostbite. They're apt to have reddened fingers and toes that *hurt!* Toddlers who roll in the snow sometimes show up with hardened areas of red skin around their necks, where snow or ice has gotten into their snowsuit collars and injured the skin.

In severe frostbite the skin is apt to be hard, white and painless. Frequently the patient will have no sensation in the injured part, and movement may be difficult or impossible. These symptoms should make you seek professional help *after* you've warmed the injured area as described below. *(Do not* rub snow on the frostbitten skin.)

Immerse or soak the injured area in warm water quickly, continuing this treatment until the injured skin feels warm to the touch. The water should be warmer than tepid, about like a bath you would enjoy (105°F or 40°C). The soaking should last about 15 to 30 minutes.

Increased pain is a good sign. It will quiet down after a while. However, continued lack of sensation signifies a more severe injury. As soon as the part is warm, get the patient to a doctor.

13

Bites: Insect, Animal, Reptile, and Human

While one of the commonest forms of childhood injury, most bites are insignificant and require little treatment or concern. Some, however, are potentially dangerous, and a rare few are downright life-threatening.

INSECT BITES

For easy reference insect bites are tabulated below according to the degrees of danger. In this discussion we will not be concerned with the ability of insects to transmit disease. (The single exception is tick bite, which we will consider later in this chapter.)

Not Threatening	Potentially Dangerous	Life Dangerous
mosquitoes	bees	scorpions
gnats	wasps	spiders
flies (sand, horse,	hornets	black widow
green, blue,	yellow jackets	brown recluse
black, may)	ants, stinging (fire)	
fleas and bedbugs	ticks	
lice *		
scabies (mites) *		
centipedes		
chiggers		

* Special medication available by prescription. Consult your doctor.

Non-Dangerous Insect Bites

(Fig. 13-1). Remember to keep them clean and utilize

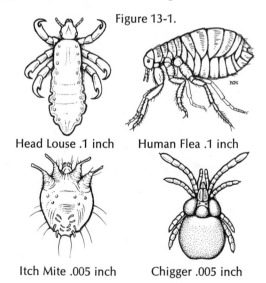

Figure 13-1.

Head Louse .1 inch   Human Flea .1 inch

Itch Mite .005 inch   Chigger .005 inch

conservative treatment to relieve itching. Frequent scrubs with a germicidal soap like pHisoHex should keep them from getting infected. PHisoHex has the additional advantage of drying, and thus hastening their cure.

Local treatment to relieve itching may include corn starch or baking soda pastes, and/or calamine lotion, a household standby for generations. Recently the use of the meat-tenderizing ingredient, Papain (papayotin), has been advocated as an amazing anti-itch preparation when made into a paste and applied to a bite. I get a mixed reaction of its efficacy from parents.

In multiple bites or particularly troublesome ones, some physicians prescribe anti-itch medications to be taken by mouth. These are usually antihistamines and may be helpful both in controlling itch and sometimes in reducing swelling. They may be tried in appropriate doses, repeated every four hours if necessary, and are most useful at bedtime.

Bites persist for a few to several days and then disappear. How swollen they get depends upon how much venom has been injected into the bite, how sensitive the patient is to the venom, and on the particular anatomical area bitten. Eyes, ears, fingers, toes, hands, feet, ankles and male genitalia are particularly prone to huge, almost grotesque swelling. Dependent areas (hands and feet, etc.) are most swollen at night and seem better in the morning. Conversely, eyes and ears are better at night, and worse the following morning. Don't panic! This is the natural history of bites and *doesn't* mean they're getting worse!

One frequent complication of insect bites of the head and scalp is secondarily swollen lymph glands. They show up anywhere on the head, but most particularly on the back of the head and neck and behind the ears. (Fig. 13-2)

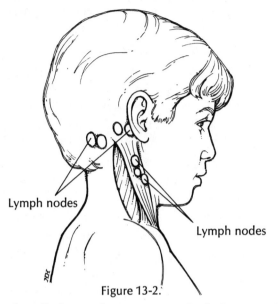

Lymph nodes

Lymph nodes

Figure 13-2.

Glands of the scalp seem particularly prominent because they have no subcutaneous tissue in which to hide, and therefore stick out conspicuously. Swollen glands secondary to simple (non-infected) insect bites are never a problem and may safely be ignored.

Prevention of Non-Dangerous Bites

Here are some ways to prevent non-serious bites.
1. Mosquitoes seem to be at their worst in late afternoon or early evening. Isn't this time to bring the toddler inside or at least on a screened porch?
2. Sometimes, when kids are swimming every day, we have a tendency to forget about baths and showers. In the summertime, when skin is exposed and constantly being "broken" by bites, poison ivy, scratches and the

like, daily bathing may be even more important than you realize. And this is a very good time to use a germicidal soap like pHisoHex!

3. In the olden days we used to rub on spirits (oil) of citronella in the hope that its strong odor would ward the bugs off. There are now much more potent, acceptable and convenient products to use for this purpose. They are especially good for small children in heavily infested areas. But beware of sensitivity—some children develop a rash after repeated or prolonged exposure to these repellents.

4. Fleas can jump from pets on to children. Fleas from pets can also infest rooms of your house. Flea collars effectively keep fleas from pets. Use them. But they do lose their effectiveness after a while. Be a sport: change them a little more frequently than the manufacturer recommends. But *don't put them on your children!* Their safety has *not* been established for children!

5. If you're in a chigger area, keep your child in shoes and well protected, with long pants and a shirt. It's not very realistic to try to keep a child out of grass entirely but that would be the ideal to avoid chiggers. This can completely prevent the chigger problem in children.

Some other assorted comments on insect infestation may be helpful. Epidemics of head lice hit the schools from time to time in *any* community of *any* degree of affluence. Your physician can order medicated shampoo which effectively *kills* both the lice and their *nits,* the little white egglike spores that are attached to the base of individual hairs.

Although it is important to remove the nits, this may

Figure 13-3.

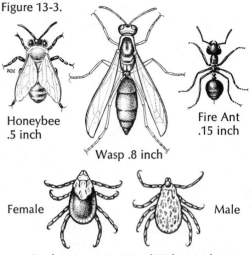

Honeybee
.5 inch

Wasp .8 inch

Fire Ant
.15 inch

Female   Male

Rocky Mountain Wood Tick .3 inch

not be easy and may require more fine-combing than your youngster will put up with in one session. But after one or two shampoos with the medicated shampoo that your physician orders, the child is *no longer contagious* and should be allowed to return to school. Some of the school laws are archaic and need to be changed! Stand up for your rights!

Potentially Dangerous Insect Bites

(Fig. 13-3). Most come from bees, and types of wasps such as hornets and yellow jackets. For our purposes they may all be treated together. The incidence of hypersensitive (potentially dangerous) reactions in *prepubertal* children is *quite small*.

I was present at a conference of approximately 35 pediatricians, in which there was over 500 years of practice available. When the question was asked if anyone had ever seen a fatal or near-fatal reaction to an insect sting *in a prepubertal child,* only one hand was raised and only one such episode could be recounted!

This is not to say that hypersensitivity doesn't occur in prepubertal children. It does, and when present it should be treated properly. But let us clearly spell out the difference between simple reaction and hypersensitivity reaction, and then most of the fear and apprehension will be put into proper perspective.

Stings from these insects hurt, swell, and sting in that order. But mostly, that's all they do! The pain may be intense, but it doesn't usually last very long. The stinger may have to be removed and sometimes this isn't easy in a jumping, screaming, hurting kid. But do it! (If you know the stinging insect was a bee, take special care to do it gently, without squeezing the entire part left behind on the skin surface. Some of what's left may be not only stinger, but also venom sac, and there's no point in squeezing the rest of the venom into the patient.)

Pain may be further alleviated by the local application of ice (the Boy Scouts used cold mud on camping trips) and a dose of aspirin. The pain of hymenoptera (bees, wasps, ants) stings always gets better in a few minutes.

Swelling in hymenoptera stings is much more evident than in mosquitoes, and may last several days. And in the areas most prone to swelling (eyes, ears, hands and fingers, feet, toes and ankles, and male genitalia) the swelling may be so great as to be grotesque.

THIS IS NOT HYPERSENSITIVITY! THIS IS NOT ALLERGY! This is still only a local reaction to the bite of the insect!

The itching comes on a little later and may be quite persistent! Local measures (cornstarch and baking soda pastes, calamine lotion, etc.) will be helpful as before. Perhaps here, even more than with mosquitoes, we have an indication to use antihistamines to relieve itching and help reduce swelling. But again, this is not allergy or hypersensitivity—just local reaction!

Dangerous (Hypersensitive) Reactions

These are not just local phenomena. The whole body, or organs far from the local site of the bite, reacts to the bite.

Some examples of these reactions are generalized hives (the most common), fainting, bronchospasm (wheezing), a feeling of the throat closing up (laryngospasm) and shock.

Any of these occurrences constitute a *genuine medical emergency*—one for which you should get professional help quickly. This is a bona fide reason for an instant trip to your doctor's office (if you *know* he's there) or to the local emergency room or hospital.

Not only will the patient need immediate care, but he should be watched carefully.

Equally important: you should prepare for the possible recurrence of such an episode after another sting. Your doctor can prescribe an emergency kit, or several of them to be kept at home, at school, etc., and carried with him when he goes to camp or takes trips.

The physician may also feel that he should begin a series of desensitization injections, so that if the child is bitten again the reaction will not be so severe. This has been proven to be very effective. We have seen many patients bitten by hymenopteran insects *after* a desensitization series, and who required no specific therapy, who did not have another hypersensitivity reaction, and therefore could be considered cured of their problem.

TICKS. Having said that I will not include diseases transmitted by insects in this section, it is necessary to mention ticks because of the publicity this little creature has received in the lay press.

Ticks are capable of carrying and transmitting viral and rickettsial (another type of microscopic organism) disease. Most infamous in this category are Rocky Mountain spotted fever in the West and rickettsial pox in the East. In addition, certain types of sleeping sickness can be transmitted from the horse to humans via the tick. While it is not necessary for you to know more about these diseases within the framework of this discussion, they are mentioned to reinforce the necessity of checking your kids and pets for ticks on a regular weekly basis.

If you find one and it seems to be "stuck" to the scalp, it is best killed, or at least paralyzed before further attempts at removal. Saturate a piece of cotton or a gauze pad with alcohol, or nail polish remover, and apply to the tick for about ten minutes. Then remove with a tweezer, grasping particularly the head part that seems fastened to the scalp. (Fig. 13-4) It should come away without too

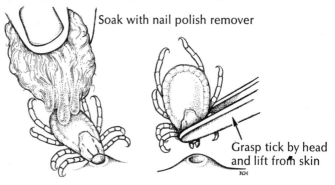

Soak with nail polish remover

Grasp tick by head and lift from skin

Figure 13-4.

much trouble, although you may take a little superficial skin with it.

FIRE ANTS. Imported from South America, these insects have become a recent threat in our southern states. This creature bites with his mouth parts, painful in itself, and then inflicts multiple stings with his tail. Although most reactions are local, systemic ones (hypersensitivity— as described above) have been noted. If fire ants have been reported in your area, find out what colonies look like and teach your children about them. And keep toddlers out of the fields and woods unless accompanied by an adult who can spot these colonies.

Life-Threatening Insect Bites

(Fig. 13-5). Three insects found in the United States are dangerous. Having had no experience with their bites, I shall relate the standard textbook information. If they

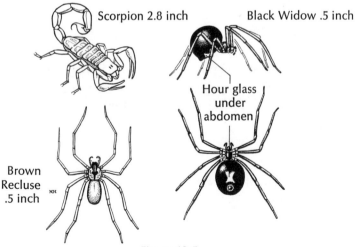

Figure 13-5.

inhabit your area, it behooves you to become further informed.

SCORPIONS. Found in the southwest. Some species produce only a local reaction, an intense, aching pain and inflammation at the bite. Others can produce convulsions, paralysis and even death in toddlers. Get help!

BROWN RECLUSE SPIDERS. Also found in the southwest and south central states. Common inhabitants of little-used closets and storage spaces indoors. They also produce a mean bite locally, and later symptoms may include fever, restlessness and a red rash. Get help!

BLACK WIDOW SPIDERS. Found all over the United States, but mostly in the southern climes. Most deadly. Yet, in the majority of cases their bites are *not* fatal. The site of the bite is sharply painful, inflamed and swollen. Systemic symptoms include dizziness, weakness, tremors, abdominal cramps and spasm, increased respirations, etc. The spider is about five-eighths of an inch across, black with red markings underneath. Get help!

ANIMAL BITES

There are two major considerations in regard to animal bites. We are concerned about treating the local wound and preventing rabies and tetanus. Let's take them in that order.

Local Treatment of Animal Bites

Again, cleanliness is next to, or even above, Godliness. You must decide whether the wound needs to be sewn, or taped closed, or needs professional help for other reasons. Understand that we are less likely to want to close bite wounds because that increases the possibility of infection. If you can't make up your mind, play this injury safe and get professional care.

If the wound is simple—most animal bites are simple puncture wounds—it should be scrupulously cleansed and left open. pHisoHex is good, and copious amounts of water will help. Frequent warm soaks—20 minutes at a time, three or four times per day—will help keep the wound open so it can drain if it wants to. Warm soaks will also help the body fight infection.

Animal bites, especially puncture wounds, have a great tendency to get black and blue. This is not, of itself, a danger sign. But increasing pain, tenderness, swelling and redness do suggest infection, and given the greater likelihood of infection with bites, these signs should make you seek help sooner rather than later.

ALL CHILDREN BITTEN BY ANIMALS SHOULD HAVE A
CURRENT TETANUS BOOSTER

The Rabies Story

Rabies is a dreaded disease. Until recently it was uniformly fatal. Nowadays, although it still carries a high mortality rate, many children with rabies have been saved. This is one disease, however, in which an ounce of prevention (shots when indicated) is worth pounds and pounds of cure.

At the present time there is very little if any rabies in pets or domestic animals in the United States. However, there is a *constant reservoir* of rabies in small wild animals and bats, and therefore vigilance *must* be maintained. There is always the chance that a rabid wild animal may bite a domestic one.

Let's make some rules about animal bites and children first, and explain them later.

1. *Notify your physician about all animal bites.* In the case of pets and domestic animals which do not come into contact with wild animals, especially if they have had shots against rabies, this is *not* urgent and may be done within a day or two.
2. *Notify your physician about all wild animal bites immediately.* The possibility of rabies infection is much increased, especially in an *unprovoked* attack, and when the animal is a bat, skunk, raccoon, fox or other small wild animal found near built-up areas.
3. *After Biting, Domestic Animals and Pets Should Be Confined and Isolated* (10 to 14 days). The appearance of illness in the animal is one of the best clues as to whether or not the threat of rabies is a possibility. *Even in animals protected by shots—obey this rule!*
4. *Wild Animals Should Be Caught or Killed If Possible* (taking great care against additional bites)! The animal will have to be sacrificed and examined for rabies. *Crucial* to the examination is the brain, so that if the animal has to be killed, spare the head as much as possible.

Having told you all the bad news, and what you urgently need to do, I can now afford to be reassuring. There are over 1,000,000 animal bites reported each year, with perhaps five to eight times as many *un*reported. Yet the number of cases of *human* rabies that occur each year (in the U.S., that is!) can probably be counted on the fingers of one hand.

However, the reason why these figures are so good is that rabies prophylaxis (a series of immunizations) is undertaken in *most* potential cases. Therefore, as mentioned before, constant vigilance *must* be maintained, because rabies is out there, in wild animals, and it *cannot* be controlled. So obey the rules and live!

SNAKE BITES

Most snakes are nonpoisonous, and their bites may be treated as simple puncture wounds. They should be thoroughly cleansed, left open, given warm soaks, and tetanus currency should be checked.

But how can you tell whether you are dealing with a poisonous snake or not? Two ways. If you have the snake you may try to identify it (see below). If you *don't* have the snake you ought to be able to tell by the wound.

Poisonous snakes leave two prominent fang marks in *front* of teeth marks of the upper jaw. (Fig. 13-6)

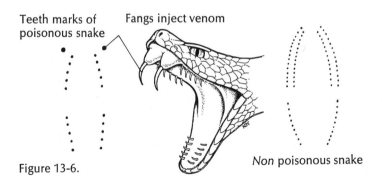

Teeth marks of poisonous snake

Fangs inject venom

Non poisonous snake

Figure 13-6.

Sometimes the fang marks are the only marks you will see. Or you may see fang marks *only* from the upper jaw of the snake and teeth marks from the lower jaw. And poisonous snakebites hurt much more than the small punctures would account for.

Treatment may be outlined as follows:

1. Make the patient recline and reassure him.
2. Inspect the wound carefully. If convinced you are dealing with a poisonous snakebite, proceed.
3. Apply a tourniquet *above* the area bitten if it's an extremity (it usually is). Not too tight. Tight enough to make the arm or leg dusky, but not so tight that you eliminate the pulse. (Fig. 13-7)
4. Make a small, single incision through each fang mark, lengthwise along the limb, and apply suction for 30 minutes if possible. Use a suction cup or your mouth if

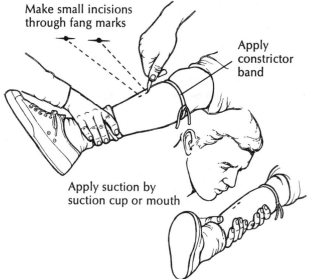

Make small incisions through fang marks

Apply constrictor band

Apply suction by suction cup or mouth

Figure 13-7.

you have no sores in it. Spit and rinse mouth
frequently during the process.
5. Ice, if available, is applied to decrease the circulation
   and thus the spread of venom.
6. Get help!

There are four varieties of poisonous snakes found in
the United States. Their illustrations (Fig. 13-8) and vital
statistics appear below. Rattlers account for most of the
bites reported, with water moccasins second and cop-
perheads and corals a poor third and fourth. Rattlers may
be subdivided into four general categories, as I've indicated. They are all worthy of your deepest respect!

Name	Locale	Habitat	Size
RATTLESNAKES			
Timber	Maine to Florida west to Texas	uplands mountains woods	1-6 feet
Diamondback	North Carolina to Florida west to Louisiana	anywhere	1-8 feet
Pacific	Washington to Southern California	anywhere	1-5 feet
Pigmy	New York and Pennsylvania west to Minnesota to Kansas south to Texas Colorado and Arizona	anywhere	1-3 feet
COPPERHEAD	Massachusetts to Florida west to Mississippi valley and down to Texas	anywhere	1-4 feet
WATER MOCCASIN	Virginia to Florida Mississippi valley and Texas	wet areas lowlands	1-3 feet
CORAL	North Carolina to Florida Mississippi valley Texas	wet areas lowlands	1-3 feet

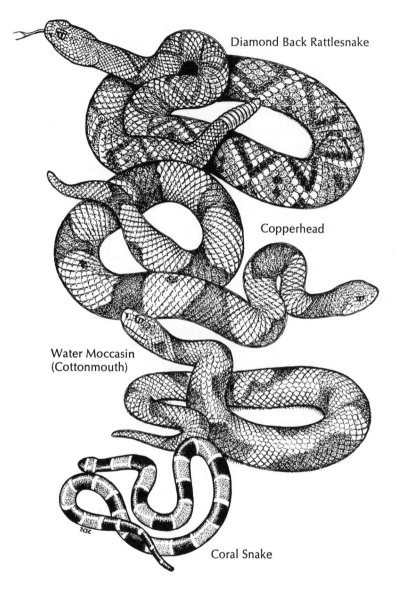

Diamond Back Rattlesnake

Copperhead

Water Moccasin
(Cottonmouth)

Coral Snake

Figure 13-8.

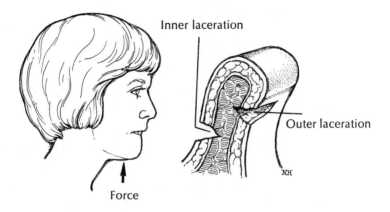

Inner laceration

Outer laceration

Force

Figure 13-9.

HUMAN BITES

The human mouth has been likened to a sewer! I'm not talking about the language that comes out of some, mind you, but rather the number and variety of potentially infectious bacteria that abound there.

Every human bite that breaks the skin must be considered potentially infected! Treat it accordingly. Wash it copiously and meticulously with soap (pHisoHex preferably) and warm water. Dry and apply an antibiotic ointment or some other disinfectant. Do not cover.

Start warm soaks for 20 minutes three to four times a day and follow each with a soap scrub and disinfectant. Watch carefully for signs of infection: heat, redness, tenderness, swelling, streaks up the arm. If any of these occur, consult your physician. Drainage and/or systemic antibiotics may be necessary.

The Self-Inflicted Bite of the Lower Lip

Occasionally a child will fall, striking his chin on some hard object and *seem* to bite clear through his lower lip. There will be a bite mark *outside* and a comparable one *inside* the lower lip, in roughly the same position. (Fig. 13-9).

Having probed enough of these wounds to know, I can reassure you that most often the bite has *not* gone clear through. The inside laceration has been produced by the *lower* teeth; the outside laceration by the upper teeth.

The *inside* laceration will profit from frequent rinsings with salt water, or a one-third hydrogen peroxide, two thirds warm water solution. The *outside* wound should receive the scrupulous care described above.

14

Drowning and Water Safety

The single most common cause of drowning is LACK OF ADULT SUPERVISION! That's the message of this chapter. If you get nothing else out of it, get that!

Hundreds of children drown every year; many of these tragedies are preventable.

In past years children used to drown in lakes and ponds, rivers and on beaches. Now, mostly, they drown in pools. We should appreciate the fact that we can fence pools, and use other devices to prevent drownings in manmade bodies of water. It's hard to fence an entire lake.

We'll tell you some ways to prevent drowning in manmade bodies of water, but the main message is clear:

NEVER LEAVE A CHILD UNATTENDED NEAR WATER DEEP ENOUGH TO DROWN HIM!

And remember, children can drown in bath tubs and

kiddy pools too! I repeat, the most common cause of all childhood drowning is LACK OF ADULT SUPERVISION! That message may save a child's life.

Let's identify the hazards, and suggest what you can do about them. The rest is up to you. (Have you really been aware of all of these?)

HOUSEHOLD DROWNING HAZARDS

1. the bathtub
2. the kiddy pool
3. flooded basements
4. homes under construction, with flooded basements, septic tanks, dry wells and water-filled depressions
5. **lack of adult supervision!**

BOATING HAZARDS

1. not wearing a life jacket
2. life preservers not available
3. sitting on the bow, where sudden shifts in course can knock them overboard. In sailing, watch the boom!
4. **lack of adult supervision!**

POOL HAZARDS

1. improperly fenced pools
2. pool without covers (adult weight-supporting) and electronic alarm systems

3. undrained pool covers (Kids can drown in six inches of water, especially in a slippery pool cover)
4. life-saving equipment not at hand (life preservers, long poles, night lights, etc.)
5. *lack of adult supervision!*
6. adults *must* remember to
   a. cover the pool
   b. drain the pool cover
   c. use an alarm system
   d. latch the gate
   e. *watch the kids!*

OTHER WATER HAZARDS

Oceans, lakes, ponds, rivers, beaches are all dangerous without ADULT SUPERVISION!

NEVER LEAVE A CHILD UNATTENDED NEAR WATER DEEP ENOUGH TO DROWN HIM!

Now I have to talk about treatment of the drowned child. This may upset the squeamish, but knowing exactly and automatically what to do in a drowning accident can save a child's life.

Listed below are ten steps to take in the treatment of the drowned child. These, and the accompanying diagrams and drawings, are a good start on your education in mouth-to-mouth resuscitation and C.P.R. (Cardio-Pulmonary Resuscitation). If you have a pool and small children—or if you live near the water—do more: take a course in C.P.R.! It's really life insurance.

At any rate, *study* this section *now!* You may not have time later!

TREATMENT OF THE DROWNED CHILD

1. No child found apparently drowned should be given up for lost. Cases have been reported of children submerged for *up to 40 minutes* (in very cold water) who have been saved! Even if you can't detect a pulse, proceed with resuscitation. Physiologic changes occur in submersion which may make the heart beat so quietly and slowly that it is virtually undetectable.

2. If possible, have someone get help.

3. Lay him on his back and prop something under his shoulders so his neck is extended and his head falls back with his chin up in the air.

4. Grab his tongue (a piece of cloth makes holding it easier) and pull it out and down over his lower teeth, lower lip and chin.

5. Clear his mouth of water, mucus, foreign matter, etc.—also with a piece of cloth—it's easier.

6. Start mouth-to-mouth resuscitation (Fig. 14-1) breathing into the child's mouth with your lips making a tight seal to his mouth. Breathe every three to five seconds (12 to 20 times per minute)—not too hard, not too deep—but enough to make his chest move.

7. Between breaths, if you are alone, shout for help!

8. From time to time, if you see his belly blowing up, squeeze down on it gently. He will burp up water and air—possibly with a loud noisy burp. Don't be fright-

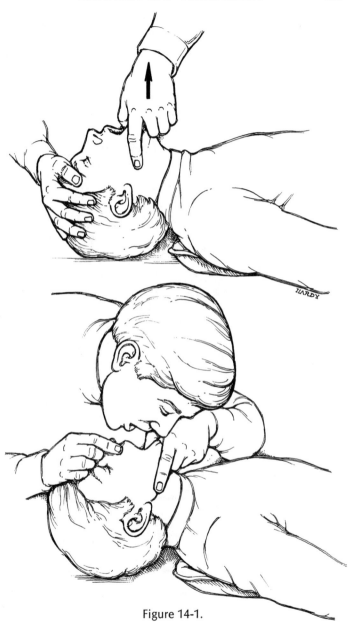

Figure 14-1.

ened. Turn his head to the side, clear his mouth of the water and mucus and continue breathing for him!

9. DON'T STOP UNTIL HELP COMES! If you lose the heartbeat, try restarting it with thumping and, whether it starts or not, begin external cardiac massage (hard pressure in the lower middle of the chest every one or two seconds) and keep breathing for him. (Obviously, you'll need help here—without it the job is very difficult.) (Fig. 14-2)

10. Read this section again, several times *before* you need it!

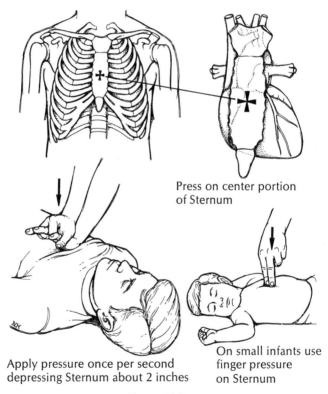

Press on center portion
of Sternum

Apply pressure once per second
depressing Sternum about 2 inches

On small infants use
finger pressure
on Sternum

Figure 14-2.

I guess we'll never completely eliminate drowning fatalities. But we can sure cut them down, and perhaps this information could prevent *your* child from becoming a statistic.

WATER SAFETY IN OLDER CHILDREN

Statistics tell us that drowning occurs most frequently among 10 to 19-year-olds, with boys making up 85 percent of the total. Although this chapter has been concerned mostly with younger children, obviously something must be said about these older boys.

Parenting becomes more difficult as children get older. But it is *not* impossible to control older children, and the statistics quoted above show the importance of the task.

You've heard it before—now hear it again. You're not your child's buddy—you're his parent. You have maturity and judgment that he doesn't have. You must insist on safe practices in water sports, in motor vehicles and in every other activity. And you'd better start being strict *early on,* so he knows that when you say it you mean it! Believe me, this can save lots of grief.

INFANT SWIMMING LESSONS

Much has been written about the pros and cons of swimming lessons for infants—and yet we still don't know whether they're advisable. Do they diminish the incidence of infant drowning? Or do they increase them? (Some people feel that if infants feel too comfortable in the water they may get into situations that they can't handle.)

We don't have the answers yet. However, the Committee on Accident Prevention of the American Academy of Pediatrics has made a recommendation. They feel that it is probably safe to begin swimming lessons with a child who can hold his breath on command. This implies a specific degree of physical capability as well as intellectual understanding, and most children cannot perform in both these areas much before the age of three years.

Whether or not the Committee's recommendation is valid I don't know. But that's what the so-called experts say.

15

Prevention of Childhood Injuries

Why can't we teach parents how to protect their children from accidents? The literature on this subject is so complete and explicit—and yet the statistics are horrifying. The *greatest killers of children beyond one year of age* are accidents and poisoning!

I can only believe that intelligent parents expect too much intelligence from their children—or that they assume the all-too-easy attitude that "It can't happen to me!"

The *really* intelligent parent must understand that if a toddler doesn't know how much it hurts to fall six feet off a stone wall, then he can't understand why he shouldn't walk on that wall! And if an intelligent parent buries his head in the sand by saying, "It can't happen to me!"—he is headed for a tragedy.

How to get the message across to you? Perhaps these true stories will accomplish that. They either happened in my practice, or in those of my colleagues. I have arranged them by age group, and in the order in which they are most likely to occur. And remember, these hazards are cumulative. The older child is subject to all of the hazards of toddlerhood, and the toddler can get into the same kinds of trouble as infants.

HAZARDS OF INFANCY (FIRST YEAR)

Falls

While Mrs. Jones's two-month-old infant was being x-rayed for a possible skull fracture, she sobbed, "I never dreamed the baby could roll over! I didn't think I had to strap him onto the bassinette for another month or so!"

Infants also fall off beds, car seats, tables and counter tops. And *mothers* fall, while carrying infants up and down stairs or on slippery and cluttered floors.

Swallowing of Foreign Objects

The morning had been a bummer, but Billy's eight-month check-up was finally over and he was in his crib for a nap. Just as Mrs. Smith was finishing lunch she heard strange gurgling—coughing sounds from the nursery. She tore up there and found him blue and choking. Turning him upside down she slapped him sharply between his shoulder blades, and the teddy-bear's plastic eye popped out of his mouth.

An older infant or toddler will put anything in his mouth! ANYTHING!

Burns

Midnight. John and Mary had been walking their colicky twins for two hours. They finally gave up and decided to have coffee. The twins seemed peaceful enough sitting up in their laps. Just as Mary started to sip her coffee (it was awfully hot!) the boy reached for her cup and it spilled all over him! John turned quickly at the scream of pain, and his dangling cigarette caught the girl in the eye!

Infants also get burned by bath water that's too hot, on radiators and hot water pipes, and near fireplaces and outdoor charcoal grills.

Drowning

Can you believe that 50 infants drown in bathtubs every year?

NEVER LEAVE A SMALL CHILD ALONE IN A TUB! NEVER!

Countless more infants drown in swimming pools. I say "countless," because the numbers increase every year as more and more private pools are built. Alarm systems, pool covers, adequate fencing, adequate marking, pool maintenance—all of these are important, but none of these is a substitute for CONSTANT VIGILANCE. (See Chap. 14)

Suffocation

As a young practitioner I thought I was brilliant when I devised a home croup tent out of the plastic bags that dry cleaning establishments were starting to use. The reports of infant suffocation from plastic bags published soon thereafter made me very humble.

Suffocation occurs even more often in choking incidents associated with the ingestion of foreign objects. And if you don't believe that this one can happen to you—when was the last time you found something in your infant's bowel movement that shouldn't have been there?

HAZARDS OF THE TODDLER YEARS (ONE TO THREE)

Burns

Dad was called to the phone while pruning the hedge with his new electric clippers. He dutifully disconnected the clipper from his new heavy-duty extension cord. Dad was very safety-conscious with little Henry around. But he forgot that the boy was teething and chewing on everything in sight—including the extension cord. Henry had to be fed through a tube in his nose for weeks while the electrical burns of his mouth were healing.

Screwdrivers in electrical outlets, dangling cords, frayed wires, space heaters, vaporizers and pot handles projecting off the edge of the stove are some of the burn hazards toddlers encounter. If there's a way to get burned, a toddler will find it!

Drowning

All of us were at the bayside beach on Cape Cod several years ago, and at least three adults were trying to keep our eyes on three children. There was an onshore breeze blowing when little Andy decided to put the rubber raft in the water and get on it. Within a matter of *seconds* he was 20 feet out, in 4-feet-deep water. He got scared and jumped off. Fortunately I had just seen him. After I got him back on the beach he was fine, but I didn't stop shaking for an hour!

Pools, pools, pools! Also ponds, streams, lakes, beaches, the surf and in older rural areas, wells and watering troughs. (See Chap. 14)

Falls

Moving into a new house is always warm work in the summertime. Daddy was really perspiring when he got the carton of books *up* the steps and into the bedroom. So he put it down to open the window and let the place air out. Danny found the carton of books to be a perfect step stool to the open window—and beyond.

Second-story falls almost always break something! Monkeys are smart enough to put three chairs one on top of another to get to the bananas—and most toddlers are as smart as monkeys. Here you need all the anticipatory safeguards your imagination can muster. Kids love to climb.

Sunburn

Blisters of the lower neck and upper shoulders (above the shirt collar), on wrists, back of the hands and the top of the feet always tattle on the parent who *thought* the child was adequately protected. There's *no way* to protect the toddler adequately from too much sun early in the season or in the tropics at mid-winter vacation time. Suntan lotions, even ultraviolet shield preparations aren't good enough. A toddler's skin just can't take as much sun as yours, so make the first few exposures brief!

Animals

A young couple, childless for several years, adopted a beautiful year-old baby. They lavished all of their attention on this new joy, apparently to the chagrin of their dog, who had been the only object of their affection for many years. It wasn't until *two* dog bites later that the parents would accept dog jealousy. This phenomenon is more common than is generally realized.

How to get along with animals is something that children need to be *actively* taught. Certain concepts should be carefully explained: leaving animals alone at feeding time, when enough playing is enough, respect for (not fear of) strange pets, and the aloof personality of cats.

HAZARDS OF THE SMALL CHILD (THREE TO SIX)

Toys

It is in this age group that toys really start becoming dangerous. From time to time a new toy comes on the market that introduces an epidemic of particular injuries. The skateboard is one of these; the injury is an explosive fracture of the lower leg and ankle. This injury is similar to the one seen when an adult jumps from a moving train and lands on his feet. I, and many of my colleagues, think that the skateboard is one of the most dangerous toys to emerge in recent years. See Appendix 1.

Burns

It was Christmas. Jennie was wearing her new organdy outfit with the puffed sleeves and long skirt. A roaring fire was burning in the fireplace, and the kids were roasting marshmallows. A live cinder caught Jennie's hemline and within five seconds she was a torch.

This story is not unusual. In India, where central fireplaces and saris have been commonplace for centuries, there are whole hospital wards of children whose burns have been sustained in this manner. They are becoming more and more common in this country. Other burns frequently seen in this age group are scalds from over-turned pots (handles off the end of the stove), electrical burns of the mouth and burns from firecrackers.

Recently there has been some concern about the

possible harmful effects of certain flame-retardant chemicals in children's clothing. Washing these clothes *three times* before the initial wearing can eliminate this hazard.

Pedestrian Safety

Jimmy ran out into the road from between two parked cars to retrieve the ball. Greg lost control of his new scooter; it plummeted down the driveway and into the street. Betsy chased her hula-hoop right into the intersection. The puppy ran into the road and Jill went to bring it back. Take your pick. They're all valid—they happen every day.

The automobile is the most lethal weapon known to man. It is responsible for the taking of more human life than all the wars of modern history. Respect for the automobile must be vigorously and indelibly impressed on every child! He must learn that every street is a minefield—constant caution is the price of survival.

For one bizarre example, never leave large boxes or cartons in the road for garbage collection. Children love to get into them, and some drivers, thinking they are empty, love to try to flatten them. This has been the scenario for more than one horrendous tragedy.

Cuts and Lacerations

Children cut and tear their flesh with knives, forks, spoons, razor blades, tin cans, broken bottles, household tools, bed frames, table corners, protruding nails, furniture handles, doorknob screws, wooden splinters, garden tools, power tools, shovels, broken toys, scissors, pens, pencils, pocketbook clasps, and on, and on, and on.

Of course it's impossible to protect a child against all of these hazards. But you can protect your youngsters from some of them by picking up, putting away, placing out of reach, and teaching safety rules.

Falls

Daddy went up the ladder. He was on the roof. Jeffrey went up the ladder. He almost got to the roof.

This is mimicry. Little boys love to do what their fathers do. And little girls love to do what their mothers do. Frequently they can't. Parents *must* anticipate these adventures and prevent them, at the expense of tears if necessary. Better an unhappy youngster than a broken one.

Suffocation

Heidi and Carl were playing hide and seek. Heidi found a large white closet in the basement with funny doors. (It was the old refrigerator.) She got into it and pulled the doors shut behind her. But it was very dark. She got frightened and tried to get out, but there were no handles on the inside. When she couldn't get out she screamed with all her might. No one heard her.

This tragedy still occurs occasionally. If you store or discard an old fridge or freezer, TAKE THE DOORS OFF!

Motor Vehicle Accidents

Children don't like to be tied down to car seats, safety belts and harnesses. One of the problems is that children sit too low and can't see out of the window. Get a pillow, raise the seat and then make your child wear the seat belt. When my children were this age, the car didn't know how to move unless everyone was buckled in! (For complete information on this subject, see Appendix 2 of this book.)

16

Prevention of Childhood Poisoning

All too frequently an older infant, toddler, or young child swallows harmful drugs or chemical compounds. Parents need to know what action to take when this happens. They also need to know about unexpected reactions to drugs and improper drug usage.

TYPES OF DRUG REACTION

Five types of drug reactions occur that need to be defined in a general way for orientation purposes.

1. *Desirable and expected*—The drug does the job expected of it when administered in the proper dosage. For example, penicillin cures streptococcal infections.
2. *Allergy*—After repeated exposure to a drug a patient may develop common allergic reactions to it, breaking

out in hives or a rash, and possibly experiencing swollen joints.

3. *Intolerance*—The patient who cannot tolerate a drug experiences side effects so unpleasant that he is unable to continue taking the medication. My daughter is intolerant of erythromycin; it gives her a bellyache. We have tried to fool her by giving her different brands in different forms, but her stomach knows. (Note that this is intolerance, not allergy.) If for any reason it were important for my daughter to have erythromycin we could probably give her other medications to relieve or even prevent the bellyache.

4. *Idiosyncrasy*—This reaction is similar to intolerance, but it is usually more severe and frequently occurs at the time the drug is first administered. A peculiarity of the makeup of the child causes the reaction. Thus, some children with bleeding problems cannot take aspirin because it makes them bleed too readily or for too long.

5. *Poisoning*—Two situations are involved here; the taking of drugs or chemicals without parental knowledge, and overdosage, as a result of unclear instructions or faulty interpretation of them.

Half the children over a year of age who die, die of accidents or poisoning. Of all children who poison themselves, the peak age incidence is about two years. And in cases of poisoning in toddlers, the most common substance is baby aspirin.

This kind of poisoning can occur even with the most careful mothers. For example, baby aspirin is kept in the locked medicine cabinet. Just as the mother is giving the toddler his proper dose of aspirin, the five-year-old comes in with a cut on his head and blood streaming down his face! Mama goes to the five-year-old, and the toddler starts eating aspirin.

In addition to aspirin, toddlers harm themselves, sometimes fatally, with substances they find all over the house: cleansers (under the sink in the kitchen and bathroom), furniture polish (in the lower cabinets), mothballs (in the bottom of closets), birth control pills and tranquilizers (in the night table), plant and animal poisons (in the garage and basement), caustics (lye and ammonia) and fuels (gasoline and kerosene).

Obviously, parents must direct every effort toward prevention (specific instructions appear at the end of this chapter). I tell my patients' parents that their houses should be "poisonproof," whether they are there or not. We all know that no mother has her toddler in sight all the time, and that's when the poisoning invariably occurs.

Poisoning occurs in the late afternoon when mother is hassled, tired and busy. On weekends. When Daddy is in charge. On vacation. When the daily routine is upset. At Grandma's home. At parties. The prevention of accidental ingestion of poisons by toddlers requires *constant* vigilance!

DIAGNOSIS OF POISONING

Most cases of poisoning are diagnosed when a parent finds an open pillbox or medicine bottle. Telltale evidence will be on the floor, on the toddler's clothing, or in his mouth. Occasionally the container will not be obvious. Some of the wilier bandits will even throw it away—they know they've done something wrong, and so they destroy the evidence. In such cases the diagnosis is made when the child develops some of these symptoms:

1. *State of consciousness.* Every pediatrician dreads cases when a toddler swallows sleeping pills. It happens time after time. The only observable symptoms may be difficulty in walking and, sometime later, sleepiness. But frequently the child goes into deep, unrousable coma. When this occurs, without any other sign, symptom, or laboratory test indicating illness, the odds are that the toddler has taken sleeping pills. Doctors may never find the source, because some parents are so overcome with guilt that they won't admit to leaving the pills within easy reach.

2. *Respiratory distress.* I recently saw an infant who was suspected of having pneumonia. He had had fever for four days and was already on antibiotics that were not doing a thing for him. When I saw him, his breathing was deep, hard, and fast (sixty to eighty times per minute). The examination was otherwise unremarkable. After he had been sent off for blood tests and x rays, my nurse asked me whether I thought the medication the mother had been giving before he got sick—three baby aspirin every four hours for four days—wasn't too much. It took us two days to wash the aspirin out of him with intravenous fluids.

3. *Vomiting and Diarrhea.* The sudden outset of very severe vomiting and diarrhea when associated with a change in consciousness could mean that the child had taken a drug or eaten the leaves, flowers, or buds of some poisonous plant. (See Appendix 3.) The clues here are the suddenness and violence of the retching and the very obvious fact that the child is critically ill.

4. *Kidney failure.* Many drugs common and rare can

affect the child's kidneys, which virtually shut down. When this occurs, sooner or later the mother notices the sparsity of urine being voided.

TREATMENT OF POISONING

This section is presented in checklist form for purposes of easy reference in an emergency. Follow the steps exactly, and in the order given.

1. Make the child vomit. There are only two exceptions here: petroleum products (gasoline, kerosene, benzene, oily substances, and cleaning fluids such as carbon tetrachloride) and caustics (lye, Drano, and ammonia). Everything else should be vomited. The best way to make the child vomit is to give him one tablespoon of syrup of ipecac. Repeat in thirty minutes if the child hasn't vomited. Please note: use syrup of ipecac. Ipecac fluid extract, a much stronger substance, should never be used. It is much too powerful, and you will overdose the child. If you don't have syrup of ipecac on hand (you should), make the child drink warm soapy water or stick your finger down his throat, holding him upside down so that he doesn't choke.

2. Identify the poison. If it's a chemical, the container should list the ingredients. If it's a pillbox or medicine bottle, call the pharmacist and find out the name of the medicine, its strength, and how much was dispensed. Then try to figure out how much was legitimately taken and how much is left or was spilled. If you can't reach your pharmacist, continue following this checklist.

3. Call for help. Try your doctor first—tell the receptionist or answering service it's an emergency, a case of accidental poisoning. If your doctor or one of his colleagues is not readily available, ask her if she knows the number of your local Poison Control Center. If she doesn't, ask her the number of your local hospital or emergency room. The local directory-assistance operator will also have these numbers among her list of emergency numbers. (These numbers should be posted prominently near your phone.)

4. Follow instructions. You may be sent to a pharmacy to get syrup of ipecac, to a local doctor's office, or to an emergency room. Take the container of chemicals, the pillbox, or the medicine bottle with you. The pills can often be identified by comparison with a pill chart, the medicine by smell.

5. If your child has taken one of the two classes of nonvomitable poisons, if the antidote is listed on the label, use it. If not, give the child bland fluids such as milk, beaten raw egg, or (if available) a suspension of charcoal. Commercial poison-control kits have ipecac and charcoal ready for use in prescribed doses, and are available from your pharmacist without prescription. They're good to have on hand, especially if your child has swiped medicine before.

PREVENTION OF POISONING

The best "treatment" for poisoning, of course, is prevention. A preparedness-action program is in order for all children, and especially for the child who has already poisoned himself once—repeaters are common. Here are some things you should do when your child is old enough to move about the house independently.

1. Get some syrup of ipecac and charcoal suspension. Put it in a convenient location, and be sure that all adults, older children, and babysitters know where it is.
2. Copy the "Treatment of Poisoning" section from this chapter and tape it to the inside of the medicine cabinet door. Keep your poison-control kit (syrup of ipecac and charcoal) here too. Make sure all medicines are properly labeled.
3. From time to time, check the contents of all cabinets that are accessible to the baby who can crawl or walk. Make sure aerosol cans, detergents, furniture polish, and other cleaning supplies are out of reach.
4. You should check the garage and basement to make sure that they are poisonproof. Be aware that accidental poisonings occur when toddlers help their parents clean or paint around the house.

Just as you learned to drive defensively, learn to think defensively about accidental poisoning. When the children are grown, you can burn these instructions along with the mortgage.

Appendix 1

Toys for Children

TOYS FOR INFANTS

Safe

Boilable teething rings
Sturdy rattles, check
 strength at seams
Brightly colored mobiles
 hung securely—in view,
 out of reach
Washable squeak toys with
 non-removable
 "Squeaker"
Stuffed dolls or animals
 that can't be pulled
 apart. Watch eyes!
Large bright balls
Blocks with rounded
 corners
Push and pull toys with

Unsafe

Sponge rubber balls that
 baby teeth can nibble on
Small objects that might be
 swallowed or inhaled
Flammable objects or
 clothing
Toys with removable parts
Stuffed animals with glass
 or button eyes
Toys painted with leaded
 paint
Toys with hidden nail or
 pins
Liquid filled items like
 teething rings or blocks—
 small leaks permit

strings or rounded
handles
Things like boxes that fit
together

bacteria to enter and
grow

TOYS FOR TODDLERS

Safe	Unsafe
Sand box	Anything with sharp edges
Buckets	Marbles
Large spoons or shovels without sharp edges	Beads
	Coins
Peg board with large parts	Games with small parts
Wooden animals (non-toxic paint)	Toys that can be pulled apart by curious toddlers
Sturdy cars and wagons to push around	Ride-on vehicles that tip easily
Large crayons	Flammable materials, clothes, etc.
Small chair and table—not for climbing	Brittle plastics
Tip-proof kiddie cars	Electrical toys
Tricycles	Toys too heavy for children of this age and size
Small broom	Objects that may break or splinter when handled roughly
Carpet sweeper	
Toy mower	
Toy telephone	Sharp or cutting toys
Dolls with simple wrap-around clothing	Wooden handles that might shed slivers or splinters
Trucks	
Tractors	
Cars	

Trains
Drums and other simple
   banging toys
Peg-pounding sets
Toys that look like Mom's
   or Dad's tools
Costume clothes

TOYS FOR THE OLDER SMALL CHILD

Safe	Unsafe
Pedal-propelled toys	Shooting or target toys
Ordinary cardboard boxes—not large enough for them to get in and close	Badly balanced mobile toys such as tricycles, wagons, cars, etc.
Simple mechanical construction sets	Pinching or cutting devices
Paints and paint books (non-toxic)	Objects that will readily come apart or shatter
Coloring books	Flammable objects and clothing
Large crayons	Electrical toys not UL * approved
Paper	
Non-toxic paste	Unsafe throwing objects (like boomerangs)
Construction paper	Tools too advanced for child use
Skipping ropes	
Modeling clay	Toys too taxing of physical strength *or* mental capacity
Paper doll sets with blunt scissors	
Cars and trucks	Model kits with many parts and complicated
Sleds	

Carpenter bench
Light, well-built tools—use
    must be taught and then
    supervised
Sturdy roller skates
Kites
Things with which to play
    store, bank, filling
    station, etc.
Playground equipment
Tire rope swing
Puzzles and games
Bicycles
Artist's set

instructions
Skateboards

* Underwriter Laboratories

Appendix 2

Motor Vehicle Safety

The following section is reprinted in its entirety from Jay M. Arena, M.D., *Your Child and Household Safety.** It is an excellent compendium of approved car seats and harnesses.

CAR SAFETY

Car Seats

Every year about one thousand children under the age of five are killed riding in automobiles. Many more are permanently disabled. Innumerable studies have shown seat belts or devices to be the single most effective safety measure presently available. Mother's lap is not safe. Children's car seats are available at major department stores and are now required to meet government safety specifications. (Make sure that the label states that the

---

* Jay M. Arena, *Your Child and Household Safety* (Washington, DC: Chemical Specialties Manufacturers Association, 1975).

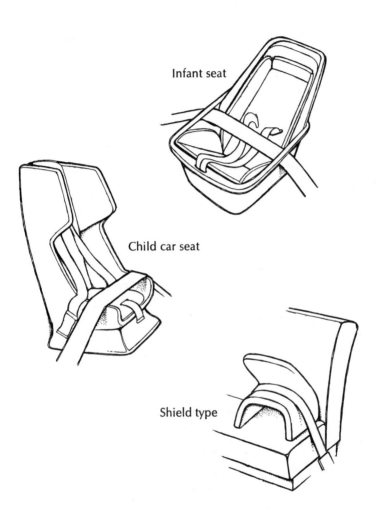

Infant seat

Child car seat

Shield type

Figure AP-2-1.

device meets Motor Vehicle Safety Standard No. 213; this is the minimum standard that may well be exceeded by some manufacturers.)

A choice should be made based on strength of construction, firmness and thickness of padding, and convenience of use. A harness unit should have a strap secured at the base of the seat to position between the child's legs. Devices that do not raise the child appreciably above the level of the car seat are preferable to those of a high pedestal.

TOT-GUARD (Ford Motors). For children 21 to 50 pounds; consists of a cushion, and foam-lined plastic shield that is placed over the child and secured with a lap belt. (An additional firm cushion may be placed under the child if necessary.)

INFANT CARRIER (General Motors). For infants not yet able to sit up; a deep container of one-piece molded plastic. The child rides backward (facing his mother). This position has considerable safety merit. A very young baby will need wrapping and cushioning to keep him positioned comfortably. Presently not subject to Federal regulations.

KLIPPAN SAFETY SEAT (Klippan of North America). For children 17 to 44 pounds; a seat of one-piece molded fiber-glass, lined with firm padding; made in Sweden. Illustrated brochure and order blank from Klippan of North America, P. O. Box 552, Chatham, New Jersey 07928. This seat has been crash-tested in Sweden where it is widely used.

SAFE CAR SEAT. A new car seat for young children (American Safety Seat, marketed by Swyngomatic) features a shield to protect the pelvis, shoulder straps, and elevation for an unobstructed view. Made in one piece, the polypropylene shell has foam padding and a safety belt gripper to prevent sideways movement. A simple buckle that can be operated with one hand gets the child in and out with ease, but the push button release is impossible for the child to use. The safety belt comes with a hook that is permanently attached to the back seat of the car, but when used in the front, the child's seat is attached to a rear safety belt.

Harnesses

Effective harnesses are available at automotive accessories and some department stores. (A label must state that the harness complies with Motor Vehicle Standard No. 209, Type 3.) A harness that keeps the child firmly seated is safer than one that allows freedom of movement.

Children over four years of age should be placed on a firm cushion and strapped in with a standard lap belt while sitting upright against the back of the seat. The cushion serves to position the belt at the correct angle across the child's hips. The belt must not be permitted to ride up across the child's abdomen.

NEVER strap two children into one belt. A shoulder belt should be used as soon as the child is tall enough (consult your car manual).

If a car bed is preferred (experts favor the Infant Carrier) choose one that is deep, well padded, and of strong construction. It should be placed on the seat (preferably the rear) with the child's head toward the center of the vehicle, away from the door. A nylon net should be stretched over the bed, and tucked firmly underneath. The bed must then be secured with two vehicle lap belts.

The best devices cannot perform its function unless installed and used according to the manufacturer's instructions. Harness must be carefully adjusted to fit the wearer. The vehicle lap belt must always be used to secure a seating device.

The back seat is safer than the front; the center of the vehicle is safer than the sides. Car seats and seat backs must lock into position if they are to accommodate a child restrained by a safety device.

AUTHOR'S NOTE

Subsequent to publication of this monograph, several excellent infant and child car seats and harnesses have come on the market, and some of the ones listed above may be unavailable. Fig. Ap 2-1 illustrates representative examples.

The reader may be assured of the safety of car seats if they are marked in compliance with Federal Vehicle Safety Standard No. 213. Harnesses are still governed by the Safety Standard listed in the text.

JGS

Appendix 3

Poisonous Plants

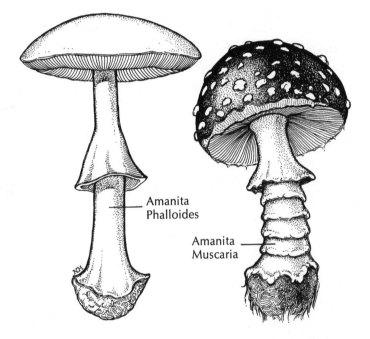

Amanita
Phalloides

Amanita
Muscaria

Figure AP-3-1.

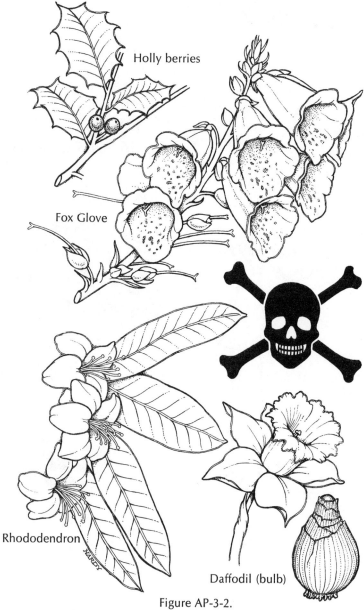

Holly berries

Fox Glove

Rhododendron

Daffodil (bulb)

Figure AP-3-2.

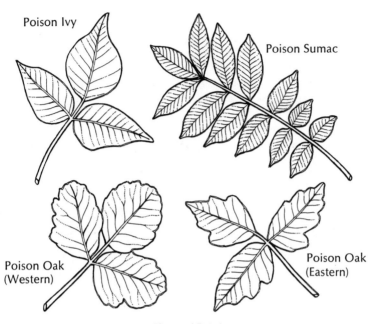

Poison Ivy

Poison Sumac

Poison Oak
(Western)

Poison Oak
(Eastern)

Figure AP-3-3.

Index